CHILD PERSONALITY AND PSYCHOPATHOLOGY: CURRENT TOPICS

CHILD PERSONALITY
AND PSYCHOPATHOLOGY:
CURRENT TOPICS

VOLUME 1

Edited by

ANTHONY DAVIDS, Ph.D
Brown University

A WILEY-INTERSCIENCE PUBLICATION
JOHN WILEY & SONS, New York ● London ● Syndey ● Toronto

An Interscience ® Publication

Copyright © 1974, by John Wiley & Sons, Inc.

Library of Congress Catalogue Card Number: 74–7030

ISBN 0–471–19696–7

Printed in the United States of America.

10 9 8 7 6 5 4 3 2 1

Contributors

Curtis L. Barrett, Child Psychiatry Research Center, University of Louisville Medical School, Louisville, Kentucky

Henry B. Biller, Department of Psychology, University of Rhode Island, Kingston, Rhode Island

Leonard D. Eron, Department of Psychology, University of Illinois at Chicago Circle, Chicago, Illinois

Edward Hampe, Child Psychiatry Research Center, University of Louisville Medical School, Louisville, Kentucky

L. Rowell Huesmann, Department of Psychology, University of Illinois at Chicago Circle, Chicago, Illinois

Monroe M. Lefkowitz, New York State Department of Mental Hygiene

O. Ivar Lovaas, Department of Psychology, University of California, Los Angeles, California

Lovick C. Miller, Child Psychiatry Research Center, University of Louisville Medical School, Louisville, Kentucky

Bernard Rimland, Institute for Child Behavior Research, San Diego, California

Eric Schopler, Department of Psychiatry, University of North Carolina Medical School, Chapel Hill, North Carolina

Judith Stevens-Long, Department of Psychology, California State University, Los Angeles, California

Leopold O. Walder, Organization for Research in Behavioral Sciences, Greenbelt, Maryland

Preface

The purpose of this series of edited volumes is to show the progress being made in the understanding of personality and psychopathology in children and youth. It presents topics of current interest to clinicians and theoreticians, and includes reports of work being conducted on the frontiers of psychological, educational, and psychiatric research. These books are designed as reference sources for researchers, educational reading for academicians and members of the helping professions, and texts for advanced students in courses on child psychology, personality, and abnormal psychology.

Each volume consists of original papers prepared especially for these purposes. Most of the papers are largely empirical, describing research projects and presenting findings from these projects. Other papers, however, present integrative reviews of relevant literature or critical evaluations of significant issues within this broad field. Over a period of years this series will publish papers devoted to most of the topical areas found in conventional textbooks on psychopathology of childhood. For example, among them are papers devoted to aspects of psychiatric diagnosis and classification, psychological assessment, learning disorders, hyperkinesis, delinquency, mental retardation, psychosomatic disorders, neuroses, and psychoses. The effectiveness of various forms of treatment are also considered, including residential treatment, special education, psychotherapy, family therapy, behavior therapy, and drug therapy. Naturally, such an extensive array of significant topics cannot be considered within the confines of any single volume. Some topics will appear repeatedly in succeeding volumes, but with new contributions prepared by different authors. Within any one volume, a given topic or issue may be covered by more than one contributor, but with different foci, methods, and/or findings.

The exact nature and contents of each volume depends on the timeliness and significance of topics and the progress currently being made by scholars and researchers. Many of the papers are highly controversial, and all of them focus on problems that are far from adequately resolved. These presentations are not designed primarily to settle issues or to provide only proven facts and final answers. Rather, they are intended to stimulate critical thinking, and to present a panoramic view of the wide terrain in great need of future creative thought

vii

and, even more important, much hard empirical work in the years ahead.

Whatever heuristic value and scholarly significance these volumes are found to have will depend essentially upon the calibre of the works submitted by the individual authors who accept my invitation to contribute papers. As editor of this series, I am indebted to these authors, all of whom are vigorous workers in varied academic and clinical settings. The papers appear over the names of those who wrote them; thus it is not necessary to mention them again here. I would, however, like to express my deep appreciation to Gardner Spungin who encouraged me to embark upon this undertaking, and to Walter Maytham, Editor at Wiley-Interscience, who helped me to complete Volume I and then move along to topics for the future.

ANTHONY DAVIDS

March 1974
Providence, Rhode Island

Contents

CHILD PERSONALITY AND PSYCHOPATHOLOGY: CURRENT TOPICS

INTRODUCTION

The present volume, which is the first in a planned series of periodic publications, includes six papers written by leading authorities on various aspects of child personality and psychopathology. These original contributions are grouped under the two categories of "Personality Development and Disorders" and "Childhood Psychoses."

In Part I, the first chapter by Henry Biller focuses on the effects of paternal deprivation on personality development and cognition, with special emphasis on academic achievement of children who have been deprived of normal father–child relations. Biller stresses the importance of "role models" in healthy psychosocial development of children and, in this regard, deplores the relative absence of "father-figures" in elementary schools. Traditionally throughout the history of elementary education in this country women have been trained to teach young children. In fact, in many elementary schools one sees no adult males other than the janitor and/or the principal. Since the occupants of these two roles have little to do with the actual teaching of reading, writing, and arithmetic, and spend practically no time with the pupils, children who have been deprived of positive interaction with a father in their own home, spend much of the remainder of their time with female teachers in what Biller terms "the feminized classroom."

Fortunately, there are current trends toward increasing employment of male teachers to work with young school children. This one particular area in which reverse employment discrimination has operated (i.e., bias in favor of females) may well have been working to the disadvantage of all youngsters, although the most likely detrimental effect has been with father-absent boys who struggle through their early school years with no adequate male model to show them that learning, and studying, and mastering of school work can be very masculine and worthwhile activities. Who knows? Remedying this imbalance in the public educational system in the years ahead may eventually remedy such troublesome developments as learning disabilities, school dropouts, delinquency, and the long-range outcome of such unrewarding childhood beginnings—wasted lives in adulthood.

In the second chapter, Eron, Lefkowitz, Walder, and Huesmann focus on relations between learning conditions within the home when children were eight years old and their aggressive behavior at that time and again 10 years later.

1

Measures of psychopathology were also obtained at the time of the followup study, since it has been assumed that aggression has a significant effect on mental health. A particularly noteworthy finding, in view of the current controversies being waged about the potential evils of violence on TV, is the importance of models of behavior furnished by children's favorite television programs. Eron et al. report that "the hypothesis that a preference for a diet of violent television would influence aggressive behavior was substantiated by our data."

In studying factors related to psychopathology in early adulthood, these investigators found significant association with parental rejection, punishment, and identification in childhood. Two major categories of variables that had significant effects on many findings from this research were sex and social class. There were consistent differences between boys and girls in the effects of various antecedent conditions on both aggression and psychopathology. In other words, the outcomes of certain childhood happenings within the family were very different depending upon whether they had been experienced by a girl or a boy. Eron et al. ascribe these findings to differential socialization of boys and girls in our society.

Although currently strong attempts are being made to minimize the differential treatment of the sexes, results of this recently completed study show that boys and girls were being treated quite differently in most households. Moreover, even similar treatments were apt to have noticeably different longer range outcomes depending upon the sex of the recipient of the particular environmental influence.

From these brief introductory comments, it should be evident that this chapter is relevant to several interrelated current concerns. Among these are differential socialization of males and females, social class as a factor in psychopathological development, and the relative contributions of parents and TV models to the identification and behavior of children and youth in today's society. Thus this longitudinal study of relations between early environment and later maladaptive behaviors provides a unique and valuable addition to the literature on childhood psychopathology.

In the third chapter, Miller, Barrett, and Hampe present a scholarly yet extremely interesting and readable account of the history and current understanding of phobias in childhood. Included is a proposed nosology for child phobia, integrating ideas and findings from several previous studies. Also described are two original instruments developed in the course of a research program conducted by Miller and his associates—the "Louisville Fear Survey" and the "Louisville Behavior Check List." Other information that may prove useful to future investigators is presented in tables showing developmental fears at different age levels, and frequencies of various fears at different intensity levels for boys and girls. A noteworthy finding is that 69% of their referrals for study of child phobia were specifically for school phobia. Thus while children show a wide variety of fears, a terrified reaction to school is by far the most prevalent form of phobia in childhood.

Miller et al. discuss findings from many published followup studies of school phobia. Since attempts to evaluate the effectiveness of treatment of other forms of psychological disorder have been sadly lacking, one might wonder why followup studies of school phobic children are found so often in the literature. It could be that since school phobia involves a specific, circumscribed, symptomatic behavior, it is easier to assess longer range outcomes of treatment. Or it may be that therapeutic success is more often found in treatment of school phobia, and this happy finding encourages followup study. With other types of emotional disorder, it may be more difficult to focalize the psychopathology, and/or the outcome of treatment may be more uncertain. In other words, there could be two possible reasons for lack of followup studies in treatment of childhood (or adult) psychopathology. One is uncertainty about the problem behavior—not knowing exactly what is being treated or changed. The other is fear of discovering that the treatment has failed to make any significant difference in terms of long-range outcome. Of course, many alternative explanations could be offered to account for the general lack of evaluation of treatment outcome that is so characteristic of the entire mental health field. Here we wish merely to call attention to this general neglect, and to applaud the fact that studies of school phobia have in many instances not stopped with the termination of treatment but have included followup assessments.

From this chapter, the reader finds neither a single personality type nor a particular kind of parent–child relationship that is specific to school phobia. Moreover, no one theory of etiology advanced to date can account adequately for all aspects of this problem behavior. There are, however, contributions to be derived from diverse theories, including psychoanalytic, social learning, cognitive developmental (Piagetian), and transactional. These various theories, and the differing kinds of therapy that have been employed, including systematic desensitization and implosion as well as traditional psychodynamic therapy, are all given serious consideration in this thought-provoking treatise.

Part II of this volume contains chapters concerned with diagnosis, treatment, and research with psychotic children. Although in absolute numbers so-called autistic children are rare, they present many perplexing and challenging problems, and consequently have provoked great interest among members of the helping professions. Recent years have witnessed the publication of numerous books about childhood psychoses, as well as the founding of a specialized publication, the *Journal of Autism and Childhood Schizophrenia*. Even among undergraduate psychology students, there seems to be an increasing fascination with infantile autism. Fortunately, this growing and serious concern for psychotic children may lead to theoretical contributions and practical understanding well beyond what might be expected from study of relatively small numbers of cases.

As I have stated elsewhere, "As psychiatrists and behavioral scientists unravel the baffling problems pertaining to causes, prevention, and effective treatment of these severely disturbed children, they are likely to gain knowledge that will make major contributions to increased understanding of normal behavior and development [Davids, 1973, p. 208]."

At this point, I imagine that many readers will be somewhat troubled by the interchangeable use of terms such as autism, schizophrenia, and psychosis in the commentary above. Actually, these terms do not exhaust the varied names that have been used by different authorities in this field, referring at times to identical phenomena, and at others to quite different forms of psychopathology. This semantic, and theoretical, confusion has contributed to the difficulty in integrating findings from clinical and research studies conducted in widely separated centers in the United States as well as throughout many foreign countries. Although the three chapters presented in this volume also show some lack of agreement in terminology, they share common views about several critical issues and should help to point the way for future researchers.

The first chapter in this part was prepared by Bernard Rimland who is now recognized as one of the world's leading authorities on problems of childhood psychosis. He made his initial impact on this field in 1964 with the publication of his book *Infantile Autism: The Syndrome and Its Implications for a Neural Theory of Behavior*. The significance of this work was recognized by receipt of the first Century Psychology Series Award for a distinguished manuscript published by Appleton-Century-Crofts.

What are some of the major contributions made by Rimland? One of the most important is his clarification of the distinction between infantile autism and childhood schizophrenia. Rimland presented abundant evidence of marked differences revealed in regard to onset and course, health and appearance, electroencephalography (EEG), physical responsiveness, human relatedness, hallucinations, motor skills, language, special abilities, and family backgrounds. As an aid toward accurate differential diagnosis, Rimland developed a Diagnostic Check List, which is completed by the parents, and provides objective scores indicating whether the child's disorder is more characteristic of autism or of schizophrenia. In the present chapter, Rimland describes recent revisions of this instrument and states his latest thoughts about these diagnostic terms.

In most clinical settings this is still a very murky area in which children who show a wide variety of severe psychological abnormalities, intellectual deficits, and neurological impairments tend to be lumped into undifferentiated groups, but with the uniform diagnostic label of "autistic." Rimland, however, is continuing his efforts to get others to recognize the crucial importance of differential diagnosis and differential treatment of children who are truly autistic, schizophrenic, or neither. At this point, many clinicians and investigators prefer to use the more inclusive term "childhood psychosis" when they know they are referring to forms of psychotic disorder other than "pure" autism.

Another noteworthy contribution has been Rimland's successful attempt to counter the predominantly psychoanalytic influence that stressed the role of parental personality in causing psychosis in children. He has shown the flimsy and unreliable nature of the evidence on which this thinking has been based and, as an alternative view, has offered a neurological theory of causation. While the validity and utility of this theory have not yet been demonstrated convincingly, it has at least helped to remove the onus of being the parent of a psychotic child.

A related development with far ranging practical implications was the foundation of the National Society for Autistic Children (NSAC). Rimland provided the impetus for this movement in which parents, and many others who are concerned with the welfare of such children, have organized to promote communication, to stimulate and support research, and to advance the cause on all possible fronts. This organization holds an annual scientific meeting that is well attended by professionals and interested laymen, and publishes a periodic newsletter that is widely distributed. In many parts of the country there are now state chapters of the NSAC, with members holding regular meetings, enlisting the aid of politicians, raising funds, writing articles for the local newspapers, and demanding better treatment for children in institutions, and more appropriate educational and treatment facilities in the community. At some future point in history, in looking back on Rimland's accomplishments, it may be that the greatest advances will have come from this aspect of his work rather than from his specific theoretical or research contributions.

In the present chapter, Rimland discusses what he believes to be noteworthy research efforts in recent years. In keeping with his primarily biological theory of causation, he has searched for biochemical forms of treatment, with special attention devoted to megavitamin therapy. He also sees benefits to be gained from applications of behavior therapy and other learning approaches. Thus the kinds of research and treatment conducted by Lovaas and by Schopler, and described in the present book, are in keeping with Rimland's view of the most promising avenues to be pursued at this time. However, Rimland believes that we are a long way from mastery of these problems, and the answers may eventually come from research in areas very different from those in which attention has been focused to date.

In the second chapter, Stevens-Long and Lovaas describe a research program, conducted at UCLA, utilizing behavior therapy with autistic children. This report summarizes 10 years of data collection, including extensive followup studies of children who upon leaving the treatment program were either returned to their homes or sent to other institutions. When this research program was initiated in the early 1960s, behavior therapy was not so readily accepted and did not enjoy the widespread popularity that it does today. Lovaas' program, however, did much both to demonstrate the utility of this treatment procedure based on operant conditioning theory and to acquaint students and behavioral scientists with some of the interesting problems that await study with psychotic children.

One incident that stimulated wide spread public interest, along with heated debate, was a feature article in *Life* magazine describing Lovaas' work with these seriously disturbed youngsters and stating openly that this treatment program made use of strong negative reinforcement. Among the highly controversial procedures used to direct a psychotic child's attention or to elicit certain desirable behaviors were loud shouts such as ''No'' or ''Look at me,'' firm grasping and shaking of the child, and even a sharp slap in the face.

Working with extremely regressed youngsters, many of whom had been deemed therapeutic failures in other settings, Lovaas was able to show rather remarkable improvement with his behavior modification procedures. This demonstrated success served to quiet many of the critics, and psychologists became increasingly concerned with applications of behavior therapy. In all fairness to Lovaas and other so-called behavior modifiers, it should be emphasized that behavior therapy relies primarily on administering positive reinforcement for desirable behaviors, with punishment and unpleasant rewards being used sparingly and only when deemed in the eventual best interests of the patient.

By the mid-1960s, Lovaas and his collaborators were publishing their findings in esteemed professional journals, and a major pharmaceutical company (Smith, Kline, and French) produced and distributed a film, *Reinforcement Therapy*, in which a large segment was devoted to Lovaas' research program. In 1969, an established textbook publisher (Appleton-Century-Crofts) produced a film entitled *Behavior Modification: Teaching Language to Psychotic Children*. This color film provides an excellent documentary on the innovative work accomplished by Lovaas and his collaborators. Shown in undergraduate psychology courses in colleges and universities throughout the country, this film by now has been viewed by literally thousands of students, teachers, and members of the helping professions.

The present chapter by Stevens-Long and Lovaas reviews much of the research that formed the basis of these films and the earlier journal articles, but it also extends the coverage to include recent followup studies of longer range outcomes with psychotic youngsters, many of whom had made noteworthy progress while in the behavior therapy program. Until recently, a teacher could show the 1969 film to his undergraduate students in a course on abnormal psychology, for example, and leave them with the seemingly happy ending that showed a vast improvement in the behavior of several of the psychotic children who were filmed at the start of the program and again after many months of treatment. One could at least hope that the obvious gains and impressive changes for the better would be perpetuated in the years ahead.

Lovaas' followup studies, however, revealed that in most cases treated in the early days of the program the gains have been short-lived. When studied some years later, several of the youngsters who had been transferred to other institutions were found to be in even worse psychological shape than they had been originally. An important finding, however, was that rather brief periods of reconditioning could reinstate earlier improvements in behavior. Even more important was the realization that the only way to ensure long-term benefits is to include parents as active participants in the treatment program. Consequently, in recent years, Lovaas has been training parents to serve as behavior modifiers for their own children, and he now believes that the positive changes will be more lasting.

This chapter also describes other ways in which specific techniques and treatment procedures have been revised on the basis of their research. As Stevens-Long and Lovaas have indicated, operant conditioning theory is basically optimistic in its underlying assumption that all behavior is modifiable, thus offering the hope that even the most baffling behaviors of psychotic children will someday be understood and controlled with greater success.

In the closing chapter, Eric Schopler traces some of the sources of past confusion, and describes the shift that has been occurring from theoretical beliefs derived largely from psychoanalytic thinking to understanding based on specific information obtained from research. Beginning with an historical introduction to the field of childhood psychosis, Schopler proceeds to consider problems in classification, theories of causation, the role of parents, types of treatment, and social and ecological factors. In each of these topical areas, he summarizes the current state of affairs and then delineates what he believes to be trends of the future.

Much of Schopler's research and clinical experience has been obtained in the course of directing (in collaboration with Robert J. Reichler) a program for autistic and psychotic children at the University of North Carolina. The outstanding calibre of contributions from this research and treatment program, established in 1967, was recognized by a Gold Achievement Award from the American Psychiatric Association (APA) in 1972. In making this award, the APA selection board stated: "Education and training techniques developed in the Child Research Project at Chapel Hill, North Carolina, have helped psychotic children lead more normal lives. Parents are taught how to function as co-therapists for their child in a program at home. The success of the project has resulted in a unique state-supported program for children with a broad range of developmental and behavior disorders [*Hospital and Community Psychiatry*. October 1972, p. 307]."

Among the major contributions of Schopler and his co-workers has been the demonstration that parents are not the culprits that some psychoanalytically-oriented clinicians have made them out to be. Schopler has conducted empirical studies revealing that the parents of psychotic and other seriously disturbed children are often distressed by the fact their child is unable to live a normal life. But they do not "cause" the child's disorder. Rather, the parents themselves suffer because of the child's affliction. In fact, Schopler became so incensed with the historical tendency to blame parents for producing psychotic children, he wrote a paper, "Parents of Psychotic Children as Scapegoats," analyzing the reasons why professionals (i.e., psychiatrists, psychologists, and social workers) had chosen to portray these unfortunate parents in such an unfavorable light.

As an extension of his much more kindly view of the role of parents, Schopler has included parents as co-therapists in the treatment program. The focus is on developmental therapy, which emphasizes education and training in keeping with the child's developmental level in various areas of human functioning. The trend is toward a more structured and controlled situation that helps the child acquire skills and abilities that will permit him to function closer to normal in several important ways. Among these are the ability to relate to others, to organize activity and play, to develop communication skills, to increase body awareness, and to improve coordination. This developmental therapy program is predicated on the belief that autistic and psychotic children suffer from neurological, biochemical, or other organic impairments. This belief in biogenic causation, however, does not preclude an optimistic outlook on future approaches to treatment of psychotic children. As Schopler's conclusions make clear, he anticipates improved methods of diagnosis and treatment in the years ahead. To accomplish these goals, however, as the title of Schopler's chapter indicates, there must be "changes of direction with psychotic children."

The three papers on childhood psychosis in this volume should reveal what has been found to date by some of the leading investigators and, even more important, should clearly show the lines of treatment and research these authorities recommend for the forseeable future. Taken together, these independent but coherent contributions should serve to correct certain erroneous theoretical notions and to dispel some harmful myths that in the past have led to wasted effort and undue heartache. The challenge for the future will certainly be no easier, and the plight of psychotic children will continue to be depressing to witness. Hopefully, however, researchers, parents, and professionals working cooperatively may be able to make great strides toward understanding, accepting, and helping these most seriously disturbed children.

REFERENCE

Davids, A. *Issues in abnormal child psychology.* Monterey, Calif.: Brooks/Cole, 1973.

PART ONE

Personality Development and Disorders

CHAPTER 1

Paternal Deprivation, Cognitive Functioning and the Feminized Classroom

HENRY B. BILLER

INTRODUCTION

Paternal Role and Sex Role

Sex-role distinctions are very much linked with the way in which we define paternal and maternal roles. The mother in most societies is expected to be nurturant and sensitive, and to be expert in communications and in dealing with intrafamilial tensions, while the father is to be most competent in dealing with environmental exigencies and in solving problems which require a knowledge of the nonfamilial environment. Aside from some expected tutelege of the son by the father in some societies, there often seems to be little concern for the quality of father–child interactions. As in the general definitions of sex roles, expectations relating to parental roles appear to be of a rather rigid nature.

Men have been judged as good fathers if they provide economically for their family, but the quality of father–child interactions has not been given enough attention. The maternal role has been seen as the key process by which children become socialized. It has been argued that child rearing is an essential dimension of the adult feminine role, but definitions of masculinity have seldom encompassed fathering activities.

Given the way males and females have been socialized in our society, fathers and mothers usually have different ranges of competencies and interests. For example, fathers in our society are more apt to be assertive and independent, whereas mothers are more likely to have a high level of interpersonal sensitivity and ability to communicate feelings. The optimal situation for the child is to have both a positively involved mother and a positively involved father. The child is then exposed to a wider degree of adaptive characteristics.

Well-fathered boys and girls are likely to possess both positively "masculine" and positively "feminine" characteristics. Children who are nurturant and sensitive as well as assertive and independent usually have fathers who are actively and warmly involved with them, salient in family interactions, and encourage interpersonal competency and problem solving skills. Children who are well-fathered (as well as well-mothered) have positive self-concepts and a comfort and pride about their biological sexuality. They are relatively flexible in their interests and are responsive to others. On the other hand, children who are paternally deprived are more likely to be insecure in their basic sex-role orientations and to either take a defensive posture of rigid adherence to cultural sex-role standards or attempt to avoid gender-related behaviors (Biller, 1971a, 1974a).

The Concept of Paternal Deprivation

Paternal deprivation is a term that can be used to include various inadequacies in a child's experience with his father or father surrogate. Paternal deprivation can be in the context of total father absence or separation from the father for some extended period of time. But the child does not necessarily have to be separated from his father to suffer from paternal deprivation. Paternal deprivation can occur when the father is available, but there is not a relatively meaningful father–child attachment.

An examination of the quality of the father's behavior when he is available and interacting with his child is needed. A child's attachment with an ineffectual and/or emotionally disturbed father can also be considered a particular form of paternal deprivation (Biller, 1972a). Paternal deprivation does not take place in a vacuum. A thorough analysis must take into account such variables as the reason for paternal deprivation, the length of paternal deprivation, the sex and developmental status of the child, the quality of the mother–child and mother–father relationships, the family structure, including sibling composition, the sociocultural background, and the availability of surrogate models.

Much of the interest in the effects of paternal deprivation has come from growing concern with the psychological, social, and economic disadvantages often suffered by fatherless children. However, it is important to emphasize that father-absence per se does not necessarily lead to developmental deficits, and/or render the father-absent child inferior in psychological functioning relative to the father-present child. Fatherless children are far from a homogeneous group. To begin with, an almost infinite variety of patterns of father absence can be specified. Many factors need to be considered in evaluating the father-absent situation: type (constant, intermittent, temporary, etc.), length, cause, child's age and sex, child's constitutional characteristics, mother's reaction to husband-absence, quality of mother–child interactions, family's socioeconomic status, and availability of surrogate models. The father-absent child may not be paternally deprived because he has a very adequate father surrogate, or he may be less paternally deprived than are many father-present children.

The child who has an involved and competent mother *and* father is more likely to have generally adequate psychological functioning, and is less likely to suffer from developmental deficits and psychopathology, than is the child who is reared in a one-parent family. This generalization is not the same as assuming that all father-absent children are going to have more difficulties in their development than are all father-present children. For example, evidence indicates that children with competent mothers are less likely to have certain types of developmental deficits than are children who have a dominating mother and a passive-ineffectual father. The father-absent child may develop a more flexible image of adult men, and at least may seek out some type of father surrogate, whereas the child with a passive-ineffectual and/or rejecting father may have a very negative image of adult males and avoid interacting with them (Biller, 1971a, 1974a).

The age of onset of paternal deprivation appears to be a very important factor. Infants often form strong attachments to their fathers as well as to their mothers (Ban & Lewis, 1971; Biller, 1971a, 1974a; Pedersen & Rabson, 1969). A strong and positive attachment to a nurturant and competent father can much facilitate the infant and young child's development. Our observations have suggested that children who are able to form strong attachments to both their mothers and their fathers during infancy have more positive self-concepts and success in interpersonal relations than children who have only an attachment to their mothers (Biller, 1971a, 1974a).

On the other hand, the lack of an attachment to a father or father surrogate in the first few years of life, or a relatively permanent disruption of an ongoing fathering relationship, may have unfortunate consequences for the child. Father-absence before the age of four or five appears to have more of a disruptive effect on the individual's personality development than does father-absence beginning at a later age period. In our research, we have consistently found that boys who become father-absent before the age of four or five have less masculine sex-role orientations (self-concepts) and more sex-role conflicts than do either father-present boys or boys who become father-absent at a later time (Biller, 1968b, 1969b, 1974a; Biller & Bahm, 1971). Other data have indicated that early father-absence is more often associated with a low level of independence and assertiveness in peer relations (Hetherington, 1966), feelings of inferiority and mistrust of others (Santrock, 1970), and antisocial behavior (Siegman, 1966).

Findings from cross-cultural studies have suggested that very close and exclusive relationships with mothers in the first two or three years of life, and the relative unavailability of fathers, are associated with sex role conflicts and sexual anxiety in adolescence and adulthood (Burton, 1972; Burton & Whiting, 1961; Stephens, 1962). Some research also points to a particularly high frequency of early father-absence (before age four) among emotionally disturbed children (Holman, 1953) and adults (Beck, Sehti, & Tuthill, 1963). It, of course, may be that father-absence at different age periods affects different dimensions of personality development (Biller, 1971a, 1974a; Herzog & Sudia, 1970).

The major purpose of this chapter is to examine the relationship between paternal deprivation and the young child's cognitive functioning and classroom adjustment. Much of the material in this chapter is based on my presentation at the 1973 Nebraska Symposium on Motivation (Biller, 1974b).

Methodological Issues

Serious criticisms can be directed toward much of the research that has been conducted concerning father–child relationships. For example, investigators have often ignored variations among father-absent families and also implicitly made the tenuous assumption that father-presence ensures an active father–child relationship. Furthermore, the potential interactions of paternal influence with factors such as variations in mothering, sociocultural variables, and constitutional-genetic variables generally have not been taken into account.

Frequently the child's sex-role development has been considered a mediating link between paternal influence and cognitive functioning. For instance, sex-role inadequacies are often associated with both paternal deprivation and academic underachievement. Unfortunately, researchers have generally not attended to the complexity and multidimensionality of the sex-role development process and have usually worked with very limited measures of sex role. In this chapter, some consideration is given to findings concerning fathering and sex-role development, and to findings concerning sex-role development and cognitive functioning. However, such topics are covered only to the extent that they are relevant to the relationship among paternal influence, academic performance, and cognitive functioning. The reader who is interested in a more detailed discussion of fathering and sex role, and the many antecedents and correlates of sex-role development is referred elsewhere (e.g., Biller, 1971a, 1974a).

PATERNAL INFLUENCE AND COGNITIVE FUNCTIONING

Academic Achievement

This section includes a description of research efforts which is some way have explored the relationship between fathering and cognitive functioning. Results from several investigations have revealed an association between inadequate father–son relationships and academic difficulties among boys.

Kimball (1952) studied highly intelligent boys enrolled in a residential preparatory school. She compared 20 boys who were failing in school with a group of boys who were selected randomly from the total school population. Interview and psychological test material revealed consistently that the underachieving boys had very inadequate relationships with their fathers. Many of the fathers were reported to work long hours and to be home infrequently, or to attempt to dominate and control their sons by means of excessive discipline.

Using a specifically designed sentence completion technique, Kimball found further evidence that significantly more of the boys in the underachieving group had poor relationships with their fathers. Responses suggesting feelings of paternal rejection and paternal hostility were considerably more frequent among the underachieving boys. Projective test data also suggested that the boys had much hostility toward their fathers because they perceived that their fathers had rejected them. There is other evidence that paternal hostility and lack of acceptance is related negatively to the child's scholastic ability (Hurley, 1967).

Through the use of extensive clinical interviews, Grunebaum et al. (1962) examined the family life of elementary school boys who had at least average intelligence, but were one to two years below expectation in their academic achievement (Metropolitan Achievement Test). These boys seemed to have very poor relationships with their fathers. Their fathers were reported to feel generally inadequate and thwarted in their own ambitions, and to view themselves as failures. The fathers appeared to be particularly insecure about their masculinity and did not seem to offer their sons adequate models of male competence. Most of the fathers viewed their wives as being far superior to them, and their wives generally shared this perception. Most of the mothers perceived both their husbands and sons as inadequate and incompetent, and seemed to be involved in undermining their confidence. This study, at best, was of an exploratory clinical nature, but it did suggest some of the ways in which the dynamics of the husband–wife relationship can affect the child's academic functioning. It is also interesting to note that boys with inadequate sex-role development are often found in families in which the mother dominates the father and undermines his attempts to be decisive and competent (Biller, 1969a).

Shaw and White (1965) conducted an investigation of the familial correlates of high and low academic achievement among high school students with above-average intelligence. Adjective checklist rating scales were administered to the students and their parents who were instructed to describe themselves and other members of their family. High-achieving boys (B average or better) perceived themselves as more similar to their fathers than did low-achieving boys (below a B average). The high-achieving boys also perceived themselves as more similar to their fathers than to their mothers, but low-achieving boys did not. Among the high-achieving group, but not among the low-achieving group, father and son self-ratings were positively correlated. Such results suggest that father–son closeness and identification are related to academic achievement.

I worked with a group of high school boys who were involved in a project designed to motivate them to utilize their academic potential (described by Davids, 1972). In general, these boys had very superior intelligence, but their academic functioning was below grade level. Most of the boys were alienated from their fathers. Many of their fathers were quite successful, but according to their sons' reports were much more devoted to their work than to their families (Biller, 1966b).

Mutimer, Loughlin, and Powell (1966) compared children who were relatively retarded in their reading ability with children who were reading above grade level. Children in both groups were generally well above average in intelligence. In a task involving various choice situations, boys who were high achievers in reading more often indicated that they would prefer to be with their fathers than did boys who were poor readers. Although not statistically significant, similar differences were noted among the girls.

Both Katz (1967) and Solomon (1969) reported data that indicated a strong positive association between paternal interest and encouragement and academic achievement among lower-class black elementary school boys. Katz's findings were based on the boy's perceptions of their parents, whereas Solomon had ratings of parent–child interactions while the boys were performing a series of intellectual tasks. Interestingly, in both studies, the father's behavior appeared to be a much more important factor than did the mother's behavior.

The studies so far discussed have dealt with paternal factors and their association with academic achievement. In addition, there is evidence that the quality of fathering is related to the child's performance on intelligence and aptitude tests.

Radin (1972) found both the quality and quantity of father–son interactions strongly associated with four-year-old boys' intellectual functioning. Father–son interactions during an interview with the father were recorded and later coded for frequency of paternal nurturance and restrictiveness. The overall number of father–son interactions was positively correlated to both Stanford-Binet and Peabody Picture Vocabulary Test Intelligence Test scores. However, the strongest relationship observed was between paternal nurturance (seeking out the child in a positive manner, asking information of the child, meeting the child's needs, etc.) and the intelligence test measures. On the other hand, paternal restrictiveness (demands for obedience etc.) was negatively correlated with level of intellectual functioning. The quality of the father's behavior, particularly paternal nurturance, appeared to be more important than did the total number of father–son interactions.

In a subsequent study, Radin (1973) reported evidence indicating that the amount of paternal nurturance at the time of the initial study was also positively related to the boys' intellectual functioning one year later. In addition, a questionnaire measure of degree of paternal involvement in direct teaching activities (e.g., teaching the boys to count and read) at the time of the initial study was positively associated with the boys' intellectual functioning both at that time and one year later.

Radin (1972, 1973) also found some interesting social class differences. For the middle-class subsample, the relationship between paternal nurturance and intellectual functioning was much more clearcut. Middle-class fathers were found to interact more with their children and to be more nurturant than lower-class fathers. These findings are consistent with those of Davis and Havighurst (1946) who reported that middle-class fathers spent more time with their children in activities, such as taking walks as well as sharing educational functions, than did those from the lower class. Boys with nurturant fathers seem to become motivated to imitate their fathers' instrumental behaviors, cognitive skills, and problem-solving abilities.

Individual Differences

Correlational data do not prove that a positive father–son relationship directly facilitates the boys' intellectual functioning. For example, a father may be much more available, accepting, and nurturant to a son who is bright and performs well in school. On the other hand, disappointment with the son's abilities may lead the father to reject him, and/or the son's performance may further weaken an already flimsy father–son relationship. Individual differences in the child's constitutional predispositions and behavior can have much influence on the quality of interactions between father and child (Biller, 1971a).

Fathers are reported to be much less tolerant of severely intellectually handicapped children than are mothers (Farber, 1962). They seem to develop particularly negative attitudes toward retarded sons (Farber, 1962; Tallman, 1965). The father who highly values intellectual endeavors is especially likely to reject a retarded child (Downey, 1963). Paternal deprivation lessens the probability that the retarded child will maximize his intellectual potential or have adequate sex-role development (Biller, 1971a; Biller & Borstelmann, 1965).

In addition to being the antecedents of some forms of mental retardation, constitutional predispositions and genetic factors may be related to other types of influences affecting the father–child relationship. Father and son can manifest cognitive abilities in the same area primarily as a function of a similar genetic inheritance. Poffenberger and Norton (1959) found that the attitudes of fathers and of their college freshman sons toward mathematics were similar, yet were not related to closeness of father–son relationship. These investigators speculated that genetic factors are involved in degree of success in mathematics and can predispose similar father–son attitudes toward mathematics. However, Hill's

(1967) findings suggest that more than genetic factors are involved in the child's attitude toward mathematics. In studying the relationship between paternal expectations and upper-middle-class seventh-grade boys' attitudes toward mathematics, Hill found that positive attitudes toward mathematics were more common among boys whose fathers viewed mathematics as a masculine endeavor and expected their sons to behave in a masculine manner.

Paternal Availability

Much of the evidence concerning the father's importance in cognitive development has come indirectly from studies in which father-absent and father-present children have been compared. The first investigator to present data suggesting an intellectual disadvantage among father-absent children was Sutherland (1930). In a rather ambitious study involving Scottish children, he discovered that those who were father-absent scored significantly lower than did those who were father-present. Unfortunately, specific analyses concerning such variables as length of father absence, sex of child, and socioeconomic status are not included in his report. A number of more recent and better controlled studies are also generally consistent with the supposition that father-absent children, at least those from lower-class backgrounds, are less likely to function well on intelligence and aptitude tests than are father-present children (e.g., Blanchard & Biller, 1971; Deutsch & Brown, 1964; Lessing, Zagorin & Nelson, 1970; Santrock, 1972).

Maxwell (1961) reported some evidence indicating that father-absence after the age of five negatively influences children's functioning on certain cognitive tasks. He analyzed the Wechsler Intelligence Test scores of a large group of eight-to-13-year-old children who had been referred to a British psychiatric clinic. He found that children whose fathers had been absent since the children were five performed below the norms for their age on a number of subtests. Children who had become father absent after the age of five had lower scores on tasks tapping social knowledge, perception of details, and verbal skills. Father absence since the age of five was the only family background variable which was consistently related to subtest scores; it seems surprising that there were no findings related to father absence before the age of five.

Sutton-Smith, Rosenberg, and Landy (1968) explored the relationship between father-absence and college sophomores' aptitude test scores (American College Entrance Examination). These investigators defined father-absence as an absence of the father from the home for at least two consecutive years. Compared to father-present students, those who were father-absent performed at a lower level in terms of verbal, language, and total aptitude test scores. Although father-absence appeared to affect both males and females, it seemed to have more influence on males. Some interesting variations in the effects of father absence as a function of sex of subject and sex of sibling are also reported; for example, in two-child-father-absent families, boys with brothers appeared to be less deficient in academic aptitude than did boys with sisters. On the other hand, the father-present girl who was an only child seemed to be at a particular advantage in terms of her aptitude test scores.

In a related investigation, Landy, Rosenberg, and Sutton-Smith (1969) found that father-absence had a particularly disruptive effect on the quantitative aptitudes of college females. Total father-absence before the age of 10 was highly associated with a deficit in quantitative aptitude. Their findings also suggested that father-absence during the age period of three to seven may have an especially negative effect on academic aptitude.

Lessing, Zagorin, and Nelson (1970) conducted one of the most extensive investigations concerning father-absence and cognitive functioning. They studied a group of nearly 500 children (ages nine to 15) who had been seen at a child guidance clinic, and explored the relationship between father absence and functioning on the Wechsler Intelligence Test for Children. They defined father-absence as separation from the father for two or more years, not necessarily for a consecutive period of time.

Father-absence, for both boys and girls, was associated with relatively low ability in perceptual-motor and manipulative-spatial tasks (e.g., Block Design, Object Assembly). Father-absent boys also scored lower than did father-present boys on the arithmetic subtest. In terms of our society's standards, such tasks are often considered to require typically male aptitudes. In a study with black elementary school boys, Cortés and Fleming (1968) also reported an association between father absence and poor mathematical functioning.

The results of the Lessing, Zagorin, and Nelson investigation suggest some rather complex interactions between father absence and social class. Among working-class children, those who were father-absent performed at a generally lower level than did those who were father-present. They were less able in their verbal functioning as well as on perceptual-motor and manipulative-spatial tasks. In comparison, middle-class children did not appear to be as handicapped by father-absence. They earned lower performance scores (particularly in Block Design and Object Assembly), but they actually scored higher in verbal intelligence than did father-present children.

Lessing, Zagorin, and Nelson also found that previously father-absent children who had a father surrogate in their home (e.g., a stepfather) did not have intelligence test scores that were significantly different from father-present children. (In general, children with no father figure in the home accounted for most of the differences between father-absent and father-present children.) These findings can be interpreted in terms of a stepfather presenting a masculine model and/or increasing stability in the home. Other evidence indicates that father surrogates and male siblings and peers can facilitate the child's sex role and personality development if they are competent and effective models (Biller, 1971a, 1974a).

The Lessing, Zagorin, and Nelson study is very interesting and impressive. In many ways it is a vast improvement over earlier research in which there was an attempt to link father-absence and intellectual deficits. For example, there is more detail in the analysis of sex differences, social class, and specific areas of intellectual functioning. In general, the investigators show awareness of potential variables that may interact with father-absence. Nevertheless, a number of serious questions can be raised in regard to the methodology of the research. The investigation can be criticized because it is based solely on findings from a clinic population. Of even more direct relevance, the study has the weakness similar to almost all of its predecessors in that the variables of father-absence and father-presence are not clearly enough defined. Two years of not necessarily consecutive separation from the father was used as the criterion for father-absence. An obvious question is whether age at onset of father absence is related to intellectual functioning. There is also no consideration as to the amount of availability of father-present fathers or the quality of father–child interactions within the intact home. Similar inadequacies may account for the lack of clear-cut findings concerning father-absence and academic functioning in some studies (e.g., Coleman et al., 1966; Engemoen, 1966).

Early Paternal Deprivation

Blanchard and I attempted to specify different levels of father availability and to ascertain their relationship to the academic functioning of third-grade boys (Blanchard & Biller, 1971). We examined both the timing of father absence and the degree of father–son interaction in the father-present home. The boys were of average intelligence and were from working-class and lower-middle-class backgrounds. Four groups of boys were studied; early father-absent (beginning before age three), late father-absent (beginning after age five), low father-present (less than six hours per week), and high father-present (more than two hours per day). To control for variables (other than father-availability) which might affect academic performance, there was individual subject matching in terms of the characteristics of the early father-absent group. The subjects were matched so that each boy from the early father-absent group was essentially identical with a boy from each of the other three groups in terms of age, IQ, socioeconomic status, and presence or absence of male siblings.

Academic performance was assessed by means of Stanford Achievement Test Scores and classroom grades. (The teachers did not have the children's achievement test scores available to them until after final classroom grades had been assigned). The high father-present group was very superior to the other three groups. With respect to both grades and achievement test scores, the early father-absent boys were generally underachievers, the late father-absent boys and low father-present boys usually functioned somewhat below grade level, and the high father-present group performed above grade level.

The early father-absent boys were consistently handicapped in their academic performance. They scored significantly lower on every achievement test index as well as in their grades. The early father-absent group functioned below grade level in both language and mathematical skills. When compared to the high father-present group, the early father-absent group appeared to be quite inferior in skills relating to reading comprehension. Dyl and I also found early father-absence to be associated with deficits in reading comprehension among elementary school boys (Dyl & Biller, 1973).

Santrock (1972) reported additional evidence which indicated that early father-absence can have a very significant debilitating effect on cognitive functioning. He studied lower-class junior high and high school children and generally found that those who became father-absent before the age of five, particularly before the age of two, had scored significantly lower on measures of IQ (Otis Quick Test) and achievement (Stanford Achievement Test) that had been administered when they were in the third and sixth grades. The most detrimental effects occurred when father absence was due to divorce, desertion, or separation, rather than to death. This study also revealed some support for the positive remedial effects of a stepfather for boys especially when the stepfather joined the family before the child was five years of age.

At this point, it is relevent to note that there is other evidence indicating that early father absence can have a very profound effect on the boy's personality development, especially with respect to masculinity of his self-concept (Biller, 1968a, 1968b; Biller & Bahm, 1971; Burton, 1972; Hetherington, 1966). Among lower class boys, father-absence before the age of two has been reported to be associated with feelings of inferiority and a low level of trust and perseverance (Santrock, 1970). The early father-absent boy, especially if he is from a lower-class background, often enters school with much uncertainty about himself and his ability to succeed.

In contrast, boys who have consistently experienced high paternal availability and involvement are much more likely to actualize their intellectual potential. Highly available fathers seem to afford their sons models of perseverence and achievement motivation. The father can provide his son a model of a male functioning successfully outside of the home atmosphere. Frequent opportunity to observe and imitate his father may facilitate the development of the boy's overall instrumental competence and problem-solving skill. But a highly competent father would not seem to facilitate his son's cognitive development if he were not consistently accessible or if the father–son relationship were negative in quality (e.g., the father generally critical and frustrating in his relationship with his son).

When the father has intellectual interests, a positive father–child relationship can greatly stimulate the child's academic achievement. If the father's activity involves reading, writing, or mathematics, it is likely that the boy will develop skills in these areas. Frequent observation of a father who enjoys intellectual activities does much to further a child's cognitive development. However, if the father does not enjoy such activities, the child is less likely to excel in school.

Creativity

There may be more controversy concerning the definition and measurement of creativity than any other psychological concept. There are certainly many types of creativity and there can be creativity in any field of human endeavor.

A major problem is deciding how to measure creativity. Is creativity just a particular dimension of intelligence, an ability to generate new ideas, or must it be accompanied by some concrete act that has, at least after a certain amount of time, been judged to be creative by others? Further discussion of the meaning of creativity is beyond the scope of this chapter, but it is important to note a few of the major issues before describing available data concerning fathering and creativity.

Fathers of creative individuals have generally been found to be very well educated and to have high status occupations (Chambers, 1964; Dauw, 1966). Among parents of creative individuals there seems to be an inordinate representation of men in professional and scientific fields (Dauw, 1966; Helson, 1971). Of particular interest is the fact that these fathers are often pictured as being very autonomous and independent in their work (Weisberg and Springer, 1961). Even though fathers of creative individuals are well-educated and are in prestigious occupations, many put their independence ahead of financial security (Helson, 1971). Fathers may play a critical role in the development of creativity by being models of autonomy and independence.

Weisberg and Springer (1961) administered a wide range of creativity tasks to fourth graders with high scholastic aptitude test scores. The investigators found that children who did very well on creativity tasks (including those tasks relating to originality, ideational fluency, hypothesis development, and flexibility of thought) were likely to come from homes where the parents were expressive, undominating, and gave the child much freedom. The fathers of the creative children generally had occupations that allowed them considerable autonomy.

Cross (1966) found that adolescent males who demonstrated a high level of flexibility and imaginativeness in completing sentences had fathers who were especially warm and accepting and listened to their sons rather than imposing their own opinions. Datta and Parloff (1967) reported that young scientists generally viewed their parents as accepting, moderately affectionate, and encouraging intellectual independence. However, those who were particularly creative were more likely to perceive both their mothers and fathers as having allowed them total freedom as children.

In a study by Helson (1967) creative college women often described their fathers as having high principles and integrity. Fathers of the creative women described themselves in ways which suggested that they were more controlled, rational, logical, and calmer than fathers of less creative women. There was also evidence that high paternal expectations and values were related to competition between the creative women and their brothers.

There is more than one path towards creativity. Some individuals develop creative talents in an atmosphere fostering self-actualization while others seem to have their creativity heightened as a result of dealing with their psychological conflicts (Biller, Singer, & Fullerton, 1969). There are some studies that suggest that creative children come from homes where there is much conflict and dissension. In a study of preschool children, Dreyer and Wells (1966) found that parents of high-creative children had more role tension and were less in agreement in terms of domestic values than were parents of low-creative children. Long, Henderson, and Ziller (1967) reported that elementary school children who manifested creativity in giving novel problem solutions were defiant toward their fathers. Consistent defiance toward the father is certainly a sign of parent-child conflict but may also be related to the finding reported in other studies that parents of creative children are likely to give them a very high level of autonomy. Long, Henderson, and Ziller also found that the creative children in their study tended to model themselves less after the same sex parent. There is other evidence suggesting that fathers may be particularly significant in fostering creativity for girls and mothers for sons (Anastasi & Schaefer, 1969). Many investigators have presented evidence that creative individuals are likely to have both positive masculine and positive feminine characteristics and to have a broad range of interests (Biller, Singer, & Fullerton, 1969).

Cognitive Styles

There is a wealth of evidence documenting sex differences in intellectual functioning (Garai & Scheinfeld, 1968; Maccoby, 1966). Analytical, mathematical, spatial, and mechanical skills are generally more developed in males; whereas, females usually perform at a higher level on most types of tasks requiring verbal fluency, language usage, and perception of details, including reading. The father may greatly influence the acquisition of certain sex-typed intellectual skills in his children (Biller, 1971a).

Carlsmith (1964) made an interesting discovery concerning the relationship between father absence and differential intellectual abilities. She examined the College Board Aptitude Test scores of middle-class and upper-middle-class high school males who had experienced early father absence because of their father's military service during World War II. Boys who were father-absent in early childhood were more likely to have a feminine patterning of aptitude test scores. Compared to the typical male pattern of math score higher than verbal score, males who had experienced early separation from their fathers more frequently had a higher verbal score than math score. She found that the earlier the onset of father-absence and the longer the father-absence, the more likely was the male to have a higher verbal than math score. The effect was strongest for students whose fathers were absent at birth and/or were away for over 30 months. Higher verbal than math functioning is the usual pattern among females, and Carlsmith speculated that it reflects a feminine-global style. Results from other studies have also indicated a relationship between father-absence and a feminine patterning of aptitude test scores among males (e.g., Altus, 1958; Maccoby & Rau, 1962; Nelson & Maccoby, 1966).

A study with adolescent boys by Barclay and Cusumano (1967) supports the supposition that difficulties in analytical functioning are often related to father-absence. Using Witkin's rod and frame procedure, Barclay and Cusumano found that father-absent males were more field dependent than those who were father present. Wohlford and Liberman (1970) reported that father separation (after the age of six) was related to field dependency among elementary school children from an urban section of Miami. Their procedure involved the Embedded Figures Test. Field dependent individuals have difficulties in ignoring irrelevant environmental cues in the analysis of certain types of problems (Witkin et al., 1962).

On the other hand, evidence suggests that a close father–son relationship is conducive to the development of analytical thinking and field independence. Bieri (1960) found that boys who perceived themselves as more similar to their fathers and as having a close relationship with their fathers did better on an embedded figures test, an indication of their field independence, than did boys who were not close to their fathers.

Dyk and Witkin (1965) reported that field-independent boys were more likely to perceive warm father–son relationships in a projective story task (TAT) than were field-dependent boys. Dyk and Witkin also described the results of a study by Seder (1957). Fathers of field-independent boys participated more actively with their sons than did fathers of field-dependent boys. Father–son participation in sports, outings, and trips was more frequent among the field-independent boys. In contrast, fathers of field-dependent boys spent relatively little time with their sons. Boys who have neglecting or passive fathers appear to be more likely to adopt a global rather than an analytical conceptual style (Witkin, 1960).

Lynn (1969) hypothesized that there is a curvilinear relationship between paternal closeness and field independence. Low paternal availability, Lynn assumed, makes the boy very dependent on his mother. He speculated that moderate father availability is most conducive for the development of field independence. According to Lynn, when the father is moderately available, the boy has an outline of the masculine role but has to interact actively with his environment to develop his masculinity. However, if the father is highly available to his son, Lynn argued, then the task of becoming masculine will be very easy for the boy, and he will not develop an analytical, independent stance in interacting with his environment.

Lynn reasoned that research with Eskimo children supports his contention that high father availability actually leads to field dependence among boys. Eskimo boys spend a great deal of time with their fathers and they seem from an early age to engage in much imitation of the father. Nevertheless, among Eskimo children, boys are not more field independent than are girls (Berry, 1966; MacArthur, 1967). Lynn also cited a study by Sherman and Smith (1967) in which orphans who received full time care from male counselors were less field independent than males from normal families.

Availability of a father or father surrogate per se is not sufficient to promote independent and analytical behavior. Some data indicate that many fathers who are constantly home play rather unassertive roles in their families (Biller, 1968a). Lynn noted that the male caretakers of the orphan boys in the Sherman and Smith (1967) study performed some typically mothering functions. Unless the father's or the father surrogate's behavior has a clearly analytical-independent component, it will not directly facilitate the boy's problem-solving ability. Lynn's analysis is interesting, but available data suggest a generally positive relationship between the adequacy of the boy's analytical ability and the amount of his interaction with a salient, competent father.

It should again be emphasized that a boy can imitate a highly available and nurturant but nonanalytical father. Corah (1965) assessed the congruence between the cognitive styles of parents and their elementary school children. His results suggested that field-dependent fathers generally have field-dependent sons and field-independent fathers generally have field-independent sons.

MEDIATING FACTORS

Behavior Problems

In addition to certain intellectual skills, other abilities that are important in academic success also appear to be hampered by paternal deprivation. There is evidence that paternally deprived children have difficulty in controlling their impulses and accepting authority. Such difficulties seem to be particularly frequent among children whose fathers are continually absent. Aggressive outbursts and delinquent behavior are reported to be more common among father-absent children, especially those from lower-class backgrounds, than among father-present children. Academic success requires the capacity to concentrate, delay gratification, and plan ahead. These abilities are less likely to be well-developed among paternally deprived children than among well-fathered children (e.g., Biller, 1971a; Biller & Davids, 1973; Hoffman, 1971; Mischel, 1961).

Paternally deprived boys frequently lack a secure masculine self-concept and have difficulties in peer relationships. Such boys are usually much more interested in getting the attention of their peers than in concentrating on schoolwork. Anxiety also seems to be more intense among paternally deprived children than among well-fathered children. Lower-class boys who are paternally deprived and insecure in their underlying sex role orientations, even though they may be quite masculine in other facets of their behavior, are often very anxious and defensive about their intellectual abilities (Biller, 1971a).

The quality and quantity of the father–child interactions can influence the child's overall adjustment, responsibility, and motivation for success. Bronfenbrenner (1961) found a positive association between the amount of time fathers spent with their adolescent sons and the degree of leadership and responsibility that the boys displayed in school. Results from a study by Reuter and me indicate that both the quality and quantity of father–son relationship must be taken into account (Reuter and Biller, 1973). For example, we found that college males who perceived their fathers as both nurturant and available had very adequate scores on personality adjustment measures, whereas those who perceived their fathers as highly available but low in nurturance, or as high in nurturance and low in availability, had very inadequate scores on personality adjustment measures.

Mussen et al. (1963) reported that instrumental achievement striving was more frequent among adolescent males who had warm relationships with their fathers than among those who had poor relationships with their fathers. Cervantes' (1965) results revealed an association between the father's inadequacy and the child's not completing high school. Results from other studies have suggested that males who have been father-absent during childhood have both lower achievement motivation and less career success than do those who have been father-present (McClelland, 1961; Terman & Oden, 1946; Veroff et al., 1960).

Independence, competence, and achievement motivation can be much stimulated by an involved father. Rosen and D'Andrade (1959) found a high level of paternal encouragement among adolescent boys with strong achievement strivings. The father can facilitate his child's independence and achievement by giving him a model of effective behavior and allowing him to make his own decisions. The quality of the father–mother relationship is also very important. A man who is consistently dominated by his wife is not an effective model for his child. Several research projects have suggested that boys from maternally dominated families are overly dependent and unsuccessful in their academic performance (e.g., Devereux, Bronfenbrenner, & Suci, 1962; Elder, 1962; Smelser, 1963).

The father who is involved in his family and is viewed as a salient family decision-maker can do much to facilitate his child's personality development and cognitive functioning. The father's self-confidence, encouragement, and involvement can be significant factors in the development of the child's academic and problem-solving skills. However, in addition to being a competent model, the father must allow his child to function in an independent and assertive manner. Paternal interference and pressure can hamper the child's ability to think flexibly and independently (Busse, 1969; Rosen & D'Andrade, 1959). Paternal domination as well as maternal domination can undermine the child's competency by denying him sufficient opportunity to solve his own problems. Some research has indicated that rigid paternal subordination of the mother and child by the father stifles the boy's achievement strivings (Strodbeck, 1958).

The quality of the mother-father relationship is an important factor in the child's academic and social success at school. For example, father-mother agreement with respect to childrearing practices and educational values seems to facilitate the child's ability to develop his cognitive and interpersonal skills at school (Medinnus, 1963; van der Veen, 1965; Wyer, 1965).

Many other studies have revealed that father-absent children have a high rate of behavior problems relating to school adjustment, both academic and interpersonal (e.g., Crescimbeni, 1964; Hardy, 1937; Holman, 1953; Kelly, North & Zingle, 1965; Risen, 1939; Rouman, 1956; Russell, 1957). Unfortunately, methodological limitations make for difficulties in interpreting the findings of most studies linking father absence with maladjustment in school. For example, such studies have usually lacked analyses relating to the potential effects of such variables as age at onset and length of father absence, socioeconomic background, and sex of child (Biller, 1971a).

Sex Differences

Most of the research concerning paternal influence and the child's personality development and cognitive functioning has focused on the father–son relationship. However, the quantity and quality of fathering can affect girls as well as boys, as is evident from data reviewed here and elsewhere (Biller, 1971a; Biller & Weiss, 1970; Fish & Biller, 1973, Hetherington, 1972; Johnson, 1963). Although both boys and girls are influenced, current evidence suggests that paternal deprivation has a somewhat more negative effect on the cognitive abilities of boys (e.g., Landy, Rosenberg, & Sutton-Smith, 1969; Lessing, Zagorin, & Nelson, 1970; Santrock, 1972).

Nevertheless, there is increasing evidence that the behavior of fathers can do much to stimulate their daughters' cognitive functioning and intellectual attainment. Plank and Plank (1954) discovered that outstanding female mathematicians were particularly attached to, and identified with, their fathers. Bieri (1960) also reported that high analytical ability in college women was associated with father identification. Crandall et al. (1964) found that elementary school girls who did well in reading and mathematics had fathers who consistently praised and rewarded their intellectual efforts. The type of model that the father represents to the girl can be very important, as is suggested by Bing's (1963) findings of a positive association between the amount of reading fathers do at home and their daughter's verbal ability.

Data from a number of studies, when taken together, indicate that high paternal expectations in the context of a warm father–daughter relationship are conducive to the development of autonomy, independence, achievement, and creativity among girls (Crandall et al., 1964; Helson, 1967; Honzik, 1967; Nakamura & Rogers, 1971).

On the other hand, paternal rejection seems related to deficits in females functioning in certain types of cognitive tasks (Heilbrun et al., 1967). Findings from a study by Hurley (1967) suggest that paternal hostility is particularly detrimental to the girl's scholastic functioning. Other types of paternal behavior can interfere with a girl's cognitive development. The highly nurturant father who reinforces the "feminine" stereotype of passivity, timidity, and dependency can also greatly inhibit his daughter's intellectual potential (Biller, 1974a; 1974b).

The degree and direction of sex differences varies with respect to which age periods and which components of cognitive functioning are considered. As with other issues relating to paternal influence, there is a need for much more research. But we do know that a warm relationship with a competent father is very significant in the personality development of boys and girls. Children who have positively involved fathers develop more adequate self-concepts and are more effective in their interpersonal and cognitive functioning than are children who have been paternally deprived or inadequately fathered (Biller, 1971a, 1974a).

Sociocultural Variables

Paternal deprivation is often a contributing variable in the complex and debilitating process of cultural disadvantage (Bronfenbrenner, 1967). Father-absence appears to particularly hamper lower-class black children. Some investigators have reported that among lower-class black children, those who are father-absent score considerably lower on intelligence and achievement tests than do those who are father-present (e.g., Cortés & Fleming, 1968; Deutsch, 1960; Deutsch & Brown, 1964; Mackie et al., 1967).

With respect to such findings, Kohlberg (1966) has suggested that the relatively immature cognitive development of the lower-class father-absent child is the key factor associated with differences in the sex-role development of father-absent and father-present boys. Kohlberg proposed that sex-role development is a dimension of the general process of cognitive development. He reasoned that if father-absent and father-present boys were matched in intelligence, differences in sex-role development would not be found or would be very small. He cited the data of one of his students (C. Smith) which suggest that differences in sex-role preference are considerably lessened when father-absent and father-present boys are matched in terms of intellectual level. Other research has indicated that there is a generally positive correlation between intelligence and appropriate sex-role preferences among young children (Biller & Borstelmann, 1965, 1967; Kohlberg & Zigler, 1967).

However, there is no clearcut linear relationship between intelligence and sex-role preference. Some data suggest that intelligence, at least as measured by the usual verbal-oriented tests, may be negatively correlated with masculinity of sex-role preference among lower-class boys (Radin, 1972). Also, as individuals gain wider experiences and education, there is usually a broadening of interests so that their preferences often become less sex-typed (Biller & Borstelmann, 1967). To complicate further the situation, all aspects of sex roles are not equally affected by rate of cognitive development (Biller, 1968a; Biller & Borstelmann, 1967).

General knowledge about social norms does seem to be related to age and experience. Father-absent children, at least after they reach elementary school, are not usually deficient with respect to their awareness of cultural values concerning sex-typing (e.g., Biller, 1968a; Thomes, 1968). Nevertheless, such awareness does not appear to be sufficient to promote a positive and secure sex-role development (Biller, 1968b, 1971a). For example, even when matched in terms of intelligence and social class, father-absent boys have been found to have less secure masculine sex-role orientations (Biller, 1969b; Biller & Bahm, 1971). The sex-role-development process involves much more than the acquisition of social norms.

Socioeconomic and sociocultural variables have to be considered more carefully if there is to be a greater understanding of the effects of paternal deprivation on cognitive development. A problem in some research is the absence of specific comparisons among individuals from different social backgrounds. In particular, culturally disadvantaged groups and members of stable blue-collar occupations (e.g., teamsters and skilled factory workers) are often both placed under the rubric of lower class. Such generalized groupings seem to obscure possible relationships (Biller, 1971a). For example, the incidence of continual father-absence is much higher among culturally disadvantaged families than among working-class families. The classification becomes very difficult to untangle because a family that has been working-class may be redefined as disadvantaged or lower-class if it becomes father-absent (Miller, 1958). In a cogent analysis, Herzog and Sudia (1970) pointed out that there have been inadequate controls for income level in research with disadvantaged children. They emphasized that differences in income level between father-absent and father-present families may be more closely related to intellectual disadvantagement than is father-absence per se. They cited some studies that suggest that when family income is taken into account, there is little or no difference between father-absent and father-present children on measures of cognitive functioning.

In any case, paternal deprivation seems to be associated with much more serious consequences among lower-class children than among middle-class children (Biller, 1971a). Some research already discussed in this chapter has suggested that among father-absent children, those who are from working-class backgrounds are handicapped more consistently in their cognitive functioning than are those from middle-class backgrounds (Lessing, Zagorin, & Nelson, 1970). A general depression in academic achievement associated with father-absence has usually been found with working-class or lower-class children (Blanchard & Biller, 1971; Santrock, 1972).

On the other hand, middle-class father-absent children often do well in situations requiring verbal skills. Carlsmith's (1964) middle- and upper-middle-class father-absent group apparently was equal or superior to her father-present group in verbal aptitude although inferior in mathematical aptitude. Lessing, Zagorin, and Nelson (1970) found that middle-class father-absent children had higher verbal scores, although lower performance (e.g., perceptual-manipulative) scores than did father-present children. Dyl and I found that, although lower-class father-absent boys were particularly handicapped in their reading skills, middle-class father-absent boys functioned quite adequately in reading (Dyl & Biller, 1973). Because academic achievement, particularly in elementary school, is so heavily dependent on verbal and reading ability, father-absent middle-class children do not seem to be very handicapped.

Maternal Influence

The middle-class mother seems to influence strongly her father-absent son's intellectual development. In an interview study in a university town, Hilgard, Neuman, and Fisk (1960) found that men who lost their fathers during childhood tended to be highly successful in their academic pursuits despite, or maybe because of, a conspicuous over-dependence on their mothers. Clinical findings presented by Gregory (1965) also suggest that many upper-middle-class students who have been father-absent do well in college. Evidence reviewed by Nelson and Maccoby (1966) reveals that high verbal ability in boys is often associated with a close and restrictive mother–son relationship. Levy (1943) reported that middle-class maternally overprotected boys did superior work in school, particularly in subjects requiring verbal facility. However, their performance in mathematics was not at such a high level, which seems consistent with Carlsmith's (1964) results.

Middle-class mothers are much more likely to place strong emphasis on academic success than are lower-class mothers (Kohn, 1959). Some findings suggest that among lower-class mothers, those without husbands are preoccupied with day-to-day activities and less frequently think of future goals for themselves or for their children (Heckscher, 1967; Parker & Kliener, 1956). Compared to the middle-class mother, the lower-class mother usually puts much less emphasis on long-term academic goals and is also generally a much less adequate model for coping with the demands of the middle-class school.

In homes in which the father is absent or relatively unavailable, the mother assumes a more primary role in terms of dispensing reinforcements and emphasizing certain values. A father-absent boy who is strongly identified with an intellectually oriented mother may be at an advantage in many facets of school adjustment. He may find the transition from home to the typically feminine-oriented classroom quite comfortable. Such father-absent boys might be expected to do particularly well in tasks where verbal skills and conformity are rewarded.

Although they may stimulate the paternally deprived child's acquisition of verbal skills and his adaptation to the typical school environment, middle-class overprotecting mothers often inhibit the development of an active problem-solving attitude toward the environment. A mother who is excessively overprotective and dominative may interfere with the development of the child's assertiveness and independence (e.g., Biller, 1969b; Biller & Bahm, 1971). The psychological adjustment of the mother is a crucial factor; a mother who is emotionally disturbed and/or interpersonally handicapped can have a very negative effect on the father-absent child's self-concept and ability to relate to others (e.g., Pedersen, 1966; McCord, McCord, & Thurber, 1962). On the other hand, mothers who are self-accepting, have high ego strength, and are interpersonally mature, can do much to facilitate positive personality development among their paternally deprived children (Biller, 1971a, 1971b).

Variations in fathering can influence the child's cognitive development, but it must be emphasized that fathering is only one of many factors which have an impact on the child's intellectual functioning. Sociocultural, maternal, and peer group values are especially important. For example, among children in the lower-class, paternal deprivation usually intensifies lack of exposure to experiences linking intellectual activities with masculine interests. Many boys, in their desperate attempts to view themselves as totally masculine, become excessively dependent on their peer group and perceive intellectual tasks as "feminine." The school setting, which presents women as authority figures and makes strong demands for obedience and conformity, is particularly antithetical to such boys' fervent desires to feel masculine.

THE FEMINIZED CLASSROOM

In this section, the emphasis is on the academic and interpersonal difficulties encountered by boys in elementary school, especially in the acquisition of reading skills, which is often a focal point of conflict. Evidence relating to the feminine atmosphere of the classroom and the potential effects of male teachers are also discussed.

Much of the difficulty that many boys encounter in adjusting to the school atmosphere is related to the interaction of their inadequate fathering and the feminized classroom. Many boys enter school with intense motivation to behave in a masculine manner. However, as a result of paternal deprivation, they are very insecure in their basic sex-role orientations. Their insecurity is exacerbated because of the omnipresence of female authority figures and a general atmosphere that reinforces behavior antithetical to their expectations of the masculine role. The emphasis is on conformity, neatness and passivity. In addition, on a maturational level, the boys are often at a disadvantage in relation to girls, and this adds to their feelings of insecurity.

Reading Skills

The superiority of girls as compared to boys in terms of language development is well-documented (e.g., Garai & Scheinfeld, 1968; Maccoby, 1966). Both earlier maturation and more social reinforcement from the mother (at least in our society) seem to be involved. It is not surprising, given the positive relationship between reading and verbal development, that girls generally do better in reading than do boys.

Much concern has been focused on the fact that boys are much more likely to have reading disabilities than are girls. Compared to girls, about four times as many boys are referred to reading clinics (Bentzen, 1963; Kopel & Geerded, 1933; Marzurkrewicz, 1960).

Part of the sex difference in reading ability may be due to less visual maturity among boys (Anderson, Hughes, & Dixon, 1962) as well as to general verbal maturity of girls (Garai & Scheinfeld, 1968). Constitutionally related sex differences stemming from genetic and prenatal factors may, to some extent, account for boys' more frequent problems in impulse control and related academic problems. The situation is very complicated, in that males may be more vulnerable to disadvantaged environments than are females. For example, some evidence suggests that more males than females are neurologically handicapped because of poor nutrition and/or lack of adequate medical assistance during the prenatal period (e.g., Bronfenbrenner, 1967).

In terms of many reading criteria relating to motivation as well as ability, girls seem to far exceed boys. Girls are more interested in reading at all ages and read more than boys (Anderson, Hughes, & Dixon, 1962). Among elementary school children, girls attach more social prestige to reading and are more highly motivated to read well in class (Strang, 1968). Girls begin to read earlier than boys. By the age of six, more than half of the girls are reading compared to less than 40% of the boys (Baker, 1948). The sex differences observed in reading ability seem to be manifested throughout the elementary school years (Gates, 1961).

Sex differences in reading are reflected in interest areas as well as in amount of time spent reading. Masculine material relating to adventure, exploration, science, technical matters, and sports is preferred by boys, whereas girls are more likely to prefer books concerning family life and romance (Anastasi, 1958). A number of studies in the United States and Europe have suggested that with the exception of a strong interest in politics, boys have more circumscribed reading interests than do girls. Usually (as with their general preferences) boys' reading interests tend to be more sex-typed than do girls' (Garai & Scheinfeld, 1968).

It is interesting to note that boys in kindergarten seem to learn to read as well as girls do when programmed techniques are used (McNeil, 1964). Such techniques may be more consistent with masculine role demands for autonomy and independence. There is some evidence suggesting that boys who have clear-cut masculine sex-role preferences prior to first grade are more mature and develop better reading skills than do boys who manifest an uncertainty about their sex-role preferences (Anastasiow, 1965). In any case, girls do better when taught by teachers in small reading groups which may be a reflection of their sensitivity to adults, particularly females. It should also be noted that girls are usually much in the majority among "high" reading groups, and this factor, too, may work to discourage boys in developing their reading skills.

Also evidence suggests that teacher expectations can influence the extent of sex differences in reading. It has been reported that boys with teachers who believe that there is no inherent sex differences in reading skills read better than boys with teachers who believe that girls are more successful readers (Polardy, 1969).

Teacher Bias

Both boys and girls report that female teachers react less favorably to boys during reading instruction (Davis & Slobodian, 1967; McNeil, 1964). However, research involving ratings of teacher behavior during reading instruction have not confirmed the supposition that female teachers react in a more negative manner with boys than they do with girls (Brophy & Laosa, 1971; Davis & Slabodian, 1967).

Nevertheless, much evidence indicates that compared to girls, boys are at a general disadvantage in terms of the reactions of female teachers. Certainly if boys feel that female teachers have negative attitudes toward them, their classroom performance is probably hampered. Moreover, some studies have suggested that female teachers give girls better grades even when boys have objectively achieved a higher level of performance (Carter, 1952; Coleman, 1961; Hanson, 1959). Boys receive more negative reactions and criticisms and less supportive feedback from their teachers than do girls (Davis & Slabodian, 1967; Meyer & Thompson, 1956; Lippitt & Gold, 1958).

Fagot and Patterson's (1969) data suggest that female teachers direct most of their disapproval toward assertive and aggressive behaviors and toward activities that are usually labeled masculine. In their study of the interactions between female teachers and nursery school children, they found that teachers reinforced boys about six times as often for "feminine" behaviors as they did for masculine behaviors. Boys, as well as girls, received more teacher reinforcement when they were engaged in quiet, sedentary type activities and appeared to be generally ignored and/or criticized for relatively mechanical or rough and tumble activities. Although such teacher reaction per se did not seem to feminize the boys, the fact that teachers reacted in such a nonreinforcing manner toward masculine behavior probably led many boys to the conclusion that boyish behavior and success in school do not go together. Another study with nursery school children suggested that female teachers initiate far fewer contacts with boys than with girls; they seem to make fewer requests for information and give less information to boys (Biber, Miller, & Dyer, 1972).

Many boys spend much of their time involved in physically demanding sports activities and acquire considerable knowledge in the process. However, female teachers seldom have much interest in such endeavors, and this widens the gulf between teachers and masculine boys. Sports can also be a constructive outlet for aggressive and competitive feelings which may otherwise come out in a disruptive manner in the classroom. There is little opportunity in most elementary schools for intense physical activity, except for an occasional recess period.

Female teachers often react negatively to assertive behavior in the classroom and seem to feel much more comfortable with girls who are generally quieter, more obedient, and conforming. Boys perceive that teachers are much more positive in responding to girls and to "feminine" behavior than they are to boys and "masculine" behavior. Unfortunately the type of "feminine" behavior reinforced in the classroom is often of a very negative quality if self-actualization is used as a criterion. For example, timidity, passivity, dependency, obedience, and quietness are usually rewarded. The boy or girl who is independent, assertive, questioning, and challenging is typically at a great disadvantage. Even though girls generally seem to adapt more easily to the early school environment, such an atmosphere does not seem conducive to their optimal development. Girls need to learn how to be independent and assertive just as much as do boys.

Although female teachers may generally respond more favorably to girls, they also tend to promote restrictive, "feminine" stereotypes. Much of the elementary school reading material also depicts females in a narrow range of endeavors and often presents an image of female inferiority. Girls usually adapt more easily than boys to the feminized elementary school atmosphere, but they may suffer even more in terms of long-term effects on their intellectual development.

Sexton's (1969) essential thesis is that our educational system exerts a very feminizing influence on children and teachers. Sexton labels feminization as inducing very passive, conforming, uncreative types of behavior. According to her, masculine males are turned off by their experiences in the classroom and reject academically related intellectual endeavors. She argues that much of the reason for our high number of male problem children, of both the inhibited and the acting-out variety, is our school system. Women are given too large a role in our school system (and in child rearing) and too small a role in our other institutions. The growing tendency toward suburban living also seems to have increased the salience of a community of women and children with little exposure to competent male models.

Sexton presents extensive data that indicate that our traditional conceptions of masculinity are incompatible with success in school. Her findings suggest that the top scholars in school are all too often feminized boys. (Males who are conforming, polite, obedient, and neat are favored.) She believes that there is no basic incompatibility between a healthy masculinity and academic achievement, but that our present educational system works against such development. She is not arguing for a rigid adherence to masculine standards, but that males (and females) be liberated and be given more flexibility and freedom.

She found that boys with high masculine standards did much more poorly in school than did those with relatively feminine values. Similar to other investigators, she reported that girls generally achieved higher grades than did boys and that more boys were identified as severely emotionally disturbed (e.g., being sent to see a psychiatrist). In most specific categories of problem behavior, over 70% of the children were boys. Almost one out of four boys was either a total failure or did barely passing work (a D or F student).

Sex-Role and School Achievement

Many of Sexton's conclusions fit well with other data reported in this chapter. However, a major criticism of her research is that she did not put enough emphasis on how socioeconomic and sociocultural factors interact with sex-role development and the educational process. For example, there is no control for socioeconomic status in her analysis of the relationship between sex-role behavior and school success. Much of the relationship she finds between femininity and academic achievement seems to be due to the differences in values between working-class and middle-class individuals. It may be that, to some extent, middle-class individuals are generally more feminized (partly as a function of being more "educated") and less concerned with sex-role distinctions than are working-class individuals, but it is also true that there are social class differences in the definitions of what is appropriate sex-role behavior. For example, middle-class adults have been found to stress intellectual competence in their definition of masculine behavior while working-class adults stress physical prowess (Biller, 1966a). Sexton's sex-role measures essentially assess degree of interest in sports, mechanical, and technical areas. What is needed is a definition of masculinity with no incompatibility among physical, mechanical, and intellectual abilities.

A related criticism of Sexton's and other researchers' work is that overgeneralizations about the relationship between masculinity and academic functioning are often made on the basis of very restricted measures of sex role. For example, many investigators have used measures of sex-role preference which force the subject to choose between either a traditionally masculine or a traditionally feminine activity (e.g., being a mechanic or a librarian). On such procedures an individual cannot score both highly masculine and highly feminine; masculinity and femininity are conceived as polar opposites. There is ample evidence that, with increasing education, individuals become more and more interested in many cultural activities traditionally labeled as feminine (Biller & Borstelmann, 1967; Kohlberg, 1966). However, this does not mean that the highly educated male has to give up his masculine interests; a well-rounded person of either sex probably has both a number of masculine and feminine interests. For example, many creative and productive people have a basic sex-role security which helps them transcend rigid sex-role stereotypes (Biller, Singer & Fullerton, 1969; Helson, 1967; Maslow, 1960).

There is also considerable evidence that sex-role preference is more subject to variation as a function of increasing experience than are either sex-role orientation (masculinity–femininity of self-concept) or sex-role adoption (masculinity–femininity of the individual's social and environmental interactions). Sex-role preference measures seem more influenced by temporary life-situation factors and may be less meaningful representations of an individual's sex-role functioning than are orientation or adoption measures. In any case, research attempting to relate sex-role behavior to other facets of personality functioning should take into account different aspects and patterns of sex role (Biller, 1971a, 1972; Biller & Barry, 1971).

A further criticism of Sexton's research is that it does not deal with the issue of varying academic performance as a function of grade level. Boys who perform the best in sixth grade are not necessarily the ones who do best in high school or college. Sexton seems to make the assumption of a consistent homogeneity in the sex-role relatedness of school atmosphere and curriculum across grade level. Such an assumption is open to question (Kagan, 1964). For example, many males do better in high school and/or college than they do in the earlier grades. This may be because the curriculum becomes more "masculinized." For these same reasons, females often have a more difficult time in the later stages of their education, particularly in college and graduate school. It is again important to emphasize that females, as well as males, are restricted in their cognitive development because of the rigidities and sex-role stereotypes associated with our educational process.

Stein's findings serve as an excellent illustration of the way in which sex typing can affect the child's motivation in relation to particular areas of school achievement (Stein, 1971; Stein, Pohly, & Muellar, 1969; Stein & Smithells, 1969). In an initial study, Stein & Smithells (1969) found that children in both elementary and high school perceived reading, artistic, and social skills as feminine, and mathematical, spatial, mechanical, and athletic skills as masculine. Such results are consistent with studies concerning sex differences in abilities (Garai & Scheinfeld, 1968).

In the Stein and Smithells (1969) study, there was evidence that sex typing of academic activities was stronger among older children. Sixth graders expressed higher attainment values and expectancies on tasks that they perceived as sex appropriate (Stein, Pohly, & Muellar, 1969). Furthermore, the boys' achievement was clearly related to their expectations. The degree to which boys perceive tasks as sex-appropriate influences the extent of their involvement and achievement. Other evidence suggests that intellectual performance is higher for children when assessment is made in terms of problems that can be considered sex-appropriate (e.g., Epstein & Liverant, 1963; Milton, 1957). However, sex-role preference measures have not been found to be related consistently to specific areas of cognitive functioning (e.g., Maccoby, 1966; Stein, 1971).

In a study with sixth- and ninth-grade children, Stein (1971) focused on attitudes and expectancies concerning mechanical, athletic, mathematical, reading, artistic, and social skills. Girls tended to rate all the areas as relatively more feminine than did the boys, particularly reading, artistic, and social skills. Both sexes gave athletic, mechanical, and mathematical skills predominantly masculine ratings, while they gave generally feminine ratings to reading, artistic, and social skills.

Stein's prediction that boys would value masculine areas as important and girls feminine areas was generally supported. The findings were most clear-cut with the ninth-grade children; mathematics was the only area in which the results were not as predicted. It is interesting to note that lower-class children of both sexes perceived reading as less important and had less expectancy of success than did middle-class children. Lower-class boys seemed to have a particularly negative attitude toward reading. There was also evidence that the more that boys tended to perceive reading as feminine, the less likely they were to be motivated to read well. Unfortunately, individual differences were not examined separately in terms of social class. A particularly strong correlation between a view of reading as feminine and a lack of motivation in reading could be predicted for lower-class boys.

Male Teachers

Less than 15% of elementary school teachers are men, and the great majority of these teach in the fourth, fifth, and sixth grades. Statistics indicate that less than 2% of teachers at third grade or below are men (Lee and Wolinsky, 1973). The percentage of men teaching in nursery school, kindergarten, and in day care centers is even lower. However, some data suggest that among elementary school teachers, men are more emotionally mature and flexible in the classroom than are women. In a national sample, Ryans (1960) reported more emotional stability, permissiveness, and child-centeredness among male teachers. Arnold's (1968) findings indicated that compared to female teachers, male teachers are more objective and unbiased in assigning grades to children of both sexes. Such data could support the notion that male teachers may generally be better models for both boys and girls than are female teachers.

Some studies suggest that boys do better in reading when they have male teachers. In contrast to the sex differences reported in the United States, Preston (1962) found that among fourth and sixth graders, German boys had significantly better reading scores than did German girls. In addition, severe reading retardation was significantly less common among German boys than among German girls. Even at the elementary level, teachers in Germany are usually males. The high frequency of male teachers may be a factor in the seemingly better reading performance of German boys. It is also important to note that intellectual endeavors such as reading are labeled as masculine within the German culture (Anderson & Ritscher, 1969). The German culture may make it very difficult for girls to optimize their intellectual skills.

Other evidence which suggests the facilitating influence that male teachers may have on boys comes from a study with Japanese children cited by Kagan (1969). In contrast to the high rates of reading difficulties reported for American boys, there was no differential sex ratio in reading difficulties found for children living in a community of Hokkaido, a Japanese island where about 60% of the teachers in the first and second grades were males.

Cascario (1971) found a tendency for male-taught children to earn higher reading achievement scores than female-taught children. Children taught by males perceived teachers as reacting more positively to boys than to girls. Such data are, of course, in direct contrast to findings among children taught by female teachers. Hopefully, we can work toward a situation where all children feel that they are valued and accepted by teachers, regardless of their sex or of the teacher's sex. Some of Cascario's data suggest that father-absent children score higher in reading achievement when taught by a teacher of the same sex. Father-absent boys may be particularly responsive to an adult male model. Cortés and Fleming (1968) found that father-absent fourth-grade boys expressed greater preference for male teachers than did father-present boys.

In addition to investigations relating to reading achievement, a number of researchers have attempted to explore the effects of male teachers on various other facets of the child's academic adjustment. Unfortunately, the majority of these studies have particularly serious methodological limitations. Kyselka (1966) studied the performance of four male high school seniors in a nursery school classroom. These "male teachers" were in the classroom for 45 minutes per day for 15 weeks. The high-school seniors reported much confusion as to their role in the classroom and emphasized their concern about discipline, respect, and their own competency to deal with young children. It must be emphasized that the type of "male teachers" in this study did not have the level of competence and experience that is typical of the male elementary school teacher.

Triplett (1968) studied kindergarten and first-grade children who were in either all male classrooms taught by male teachers or in coeducational classes taught by female teachers. Both groups were similar in academic achievement. However, in terms of paper and pencil tests, boys in the all male sections had more positive self-esteem and attitudes toward school and teachers. Nevertheless, a major problem in interpreting the results of this study is the impossibility of separating out the effects of the male teacher from the all male peer group.

McFarland (1969) assigned first-grade children to one of two classes. In one class there was a supervising female teacher with 26 male college juniors who were sequentially scheduled over the school year. In the other class there was a female teacher and a female supervisor. Unfortunately in this study, no male teacher was present throughout the school year. One also has to question the perceived status of younger males in such a transient teaching position. In general, little difference was found between the two groups. The female-taught group did better in arithmetic, but both groups performed similarly in other areas. McFarland did present observations that some children, particularly boys, do well when they have a close and positive relationship with a male teacher but again the nature of this study makes any conclusions very tenuous.

Brophy and Laosa (1971) compared the behavior of children in a kindergarten conducted by a woman with the behavior of children in a kindergarten conducted by a man and a woman (husband and wife). In general, few differences were observed. The investigators found no consistent relationships between measures of the children's sex-typing as a function of whether they were taught by the male teacher. However, children of both sexes who were in the kindergarten with the male teacher performed better on tasks related to spatial skills, and boys in this kindergarten seemed to enjoy a relatively higher peer status.

The care with which Brophy and Laosa developed and selected measures of

sex-typing, the amount of data they collected, and the depth to which they analyzed their results are very impressive. Nevertheless, the fact that their investigation was limited to two comparison groups seems to greatly restrict the generality of their findings.

Lee and Wolinsky (1973) did an excellent observational study focusing on
the differential behavior of male and female teachers in classrooms with young
children. They studied teachers in 18 classes ranging from preschool through
second grade. All the classes had two teachers, and in 12 of the classes responsibilities were shared by a male and female teacher. Both male and female
teachers were more disapproving of boys than of girls but male teachers were
generally more approving of boys than were female teachers. Male teachers
gave boys much more positive reinforcement than did female teachers. Male
teachers seemed to be unbiased in their evaluation of boys but rather nonevalua-
tive toward girls.

Compared to female teachers, male teachers were more likely to allow the
children freedom in choosing activities and in forming their own groups. Male
teachers were more responsive to the children's activities, whereas female teachers were more likely to initiate groupings and activities. Male teachers were
more responsive to male activities in contrast to female teachers who were most
responsive to non-sex-typed activities. The findings regarding female teachers
are in contrast to other findings (e.g., Fagot & Patterson, 1969) which suggest
that female teachers are particularly responsive and supportive to feminine activities.

However, male teachers seemed particularly sex-biased in their leadership assignments. They gave boys leadership assignments about four times as often as
girls. In contrast, female teachers gave leadership assignments approximately
twice as often to girls as to boys.

Boys clearly preferred male teachers whereas there was no clear-cut preference regarding sex of teacher among girls. However, girls as well as boys generally perceived that their male teachers liked them better than did their female
teachers. The children attributed no sex preference to male teachers but viewed
their female teachers as preferring girls. On the other hand, when asked to name
their teachers' favorite child, boys reported that male teachers strongly preferred
boys but did not attribute a sex preference to their female teachers. Girls generally named girls as both male and female teachers' favorite children. When
these findings are combined with the observations on teacher behavior, they
lend support to the positive student morale value of male teachers, especially
for boys. This study is interesting in suggesting the possible advantages of
male–female team teaching. However, as with the Brophy and Laosa (1971)
study, one cannot draw any conclusions with respect to the advantages or disadvantages of classrooms with *only* male teachers.

Perhaps more important, there has been no systematic investigation of how
adequate the teachers in these studies were in terms of their own sex-role behav-

ior and what types of personality characteristics they possessed. The studies would have been much improved if several different classes could have been compared—some having a male teacher, some having a female teacher, and some having both a male and a female teacher. In addition, careful personality assessment of the teachers might reveal important interactions among sex of teacher, personality of teacher, sex of child, and personality of child. For example, assertive male teachers may have the greatest effect on paternally deprived boys with aggressive characteristics but have little effect on well-fathered moderately aggressive girls.

Previous studies are also limited in that the children studied are from primarily middle- and upper-middle-class backgrounds. The situation gets even more complicated when we consider the importance of sociocultural variables. For example, as emphasized earlier in this chapter, among boys who are father-absent, those who come from lower-class backgrounds are particularly likely to perform inadequately on academic tasks. A male teacher, other things being equal, may have a greater effect on lower-class children than on middle-class children. These are obviously simplified examples, but they again point out the need for more research. The systematic evaluation of the effects of sex of teacher on the cognitive functioning and general academic adjustment of children is a little explored but very provocative and promising area of research.

In a number of different educational and treatment contexts, I have observed some rather dramatic effects of paternally deprived children responding to the attention of an interested male adult. In practicing and supervising psychotherapy with young boys, I have often found an improvement in school work associated with explicit reinforcement from adult males. Some particularly interesting results were achieved by having books about sports and sports' heroes available during therapy. In these cases, reading and talking about sports became a major focus of therapy. These boys needed to become aware that there was no incompatibility between intellectual endeavors such as reading and their conception of masculine behavior. It seemed particularly helpful to the boys that the therapist clearly exhibited athletic as well as reading skill, and that, equally as important, he obviously enjoyed both reading and athletics. In therapy the emphasis was on modeling and joint participation in concretely reinforcing activities. Similarly, through the process of family therapy, positive involvement of the father (or father surrogate) has often been associated with a marked improvement in the child's academic functioning. However, clinical experiences are no substitute for systematic research.

Concluding Remarks

Our educational system could do much to mitigate the effects of paternal deprivation if more male teachers were available, particularly in nursery school, kindergarten, and early elementary school grades. Competent and interpersonally able male teachers could facilitate the cognitive development of many children as well as contribute to' their general social functioning.

There is much need for greater incentives to encourage more males to become teachers of young children. There has to be more freedom and autonomy to innovate as well as greater financial rewards. We must make both men and women aware of the impact that males can have in child development and also the importance of male influence in the early years of the child's development. Just having more male teachers is not going to be a significant factor. The feminized school atmosphere must become more humanized, and teachers must be selected on the basis of interpersonal ability and overall competency. If a man is basically feminized or allows himself to be dominated by a restrictive atmosphere, he may be a particularly poor model for children.

The remedy for the feminized classroom is not just having more male teachers per se, but giving men and women a more equal distribution of the responsibilities and decisions related to education. As Sexton (1969) suggests, both boys and girls might be better off if there were more women in top administrative positions as well as more men in the classroom. As in the family situation, children can profit much from opportunities of seeing males and females interact in a cooperative creative manner. Men and women in the classroom could help each other better understand the different socialization experiences of males and females.

Even if significantly more male teachers are not immediately available, our school system could better utilize existing personnel. Many of the males who teach in the upper elementary school grades, junior high, and high school could also be very effective with younger children. Again, we need to put emphasis on the importance of males interacting with young children (as well as with older children). Programs could also be planned so that male teachers could spend some of their time with a wider range of children, particularly in tasks where they had much skill and enthusiasm. Perhaps their responsibilities could be concentrated on father-deprived children. In addition, other males such as older students or retired men may be encouraged to participate in the educational process of young children.

There is a general need to make our schools more a part of the community and to invite greater participation especially from fathers. Men in the community could be invited to talk about and demonstrate their work. Participants could include members of various professions, skilled craftsmen and technicians, politicians, and athletes.

Of course, it is also important to have women in various occupations come to the school and describe their activities. Both boys and girls need to become aware that women can be successful in "traditionally masculine" fields.

Sexton (1969) suggests that we have more flexibility in educational job classifications. She advocates school job classifications such as resource person, group leader, or technical specialist. Such positions could be filled by individuals with skills or knowledge that would have more relevance to children. Electricians, carpenters, mechanics, dentists, politicians, plumbers, and such could fill these jobs. Individuals with various physical or interpersonal skills could also be recruited. In addition, we could recruit more paraprofessional teacher aides from the community. (Such jobs might also do much to lessen our unemployment rates.) These aides could assist in specific school subjects but could also instruct both teachers and children in certain areas.

An atmosphere in which older children help younger children or children help less able peers of the same age could go a long way toward encouraging males to gain the skills and experiences that are important in being competent fathers. Men from the community could come in during lunch breaks and eat with the children. They could also interact with children on the playground and ride with them on school buses. Hopefully, businesses and industries could regularly cooperate in giving men the opportunities and incentives to make such contributions. Another function that could be performed by business and industry would be to setup regular visits for children to various settings in their community. Such visits can be very educational and also can provide children with more experiences in interacting with competent adults of both sexes. Some of these, and other suggestions, have also been made by a number of observers who have criticized the lack of male influence in our educational system (e.g., Biller, 1971a, 1974b; Garai & Scheinfeld, 1968; Grambs & Waetjen, 1966; Ostrovsky, 1959; Sexton, 1969).

It should be emphasized that there are many practical implications which transcend our school system. We generally need a greater participation of men in child rearing and in various situations relating to adult–child interaction. Practical implications relating to family life, therapy, and other phases of community interaction are outlined elsewhere (Biller, 1971a, 1974a, 1974b; Biller & Meredith, 1974).

REFERENCES

Altus, W. D. The broken home and factors of adjustment. *Psychological Reports*, 1958, **4**, 477.

Anastasi, A. *Differential psychology: Individual and group differences in behavior*. New York: Macmillan, 1958.

Anastasi, A. & Schaefer, C. E. Biographical correlates of artistic and literary creativity in adolescent girls. *Journal of Applied Psychology*, 1969, **53**, 267–273.

Anastasiow, N. S. Success in school and boys' sex-role patterns. *Child Development*, 1965, **36**, 1053–1066.

Anderson, I. H., Hughes, B. O., & Dixon, W. R. The rate of reading development and its relation to age of learning to read, sex, and intelligence. *Journal of Educational Research*, 1962, **65**, 132–135.

Anderson, R., & Ritscher, C. Pupil progress. In R. Ebel (Ed.), *Encyclopedia of educational research*. London: Macmillan, 1969.

Arnold, R. D. The achievement of boys and girls taught by men and women teachers. *Elementary School Journal*, 1968, **68**, 367–372.

Ayres, P. *Laggards in our schools*. New York: Russel-Sage, 1909.

Baker, E. Reading problems are caused. *Elementary English*, 1948, **25**, 360.

Ban, P. L., & Lewis, M. Mothers and fathers, girls and boys: Attachment behavior in the one-year-old. Paper presented at the meeting of the Eastern Psychological Association, New York, April, 1971.

Bandura, A., & Walters, R. H. *Social learning and personality development*. New York: Holt, Rinehart, & Winston, 1963.

Barclay, A. G., & Cusumano, D. Father-absence, cross-sex identity, and field-dependent behavior in male adolescents. *Child Development*, 1967, **38**, 243–250.

Beck, A. T., Sehti, B. B., & Tuthill, R. W. Childhood bereavement and adult depression. *Archives of General Psychiatry*, 1963, **9**, 295–302.

Bee, H., Van Egeren, L., Streissguth, A., Nyman, B., & Leckie, M. Social class differences in maternal teaching strategies and speech patterns. *Developmental Psychology*, 1969, **1**, 724–734.

Bentzen, F. Sex ratios in learning and behavior disorders. *American Journal of Orthopsychiatry*, 1963, **33**, 92–98.

Biber, H., Miller, L. B., & Dyer, J. L. Feminization in preschool. *Developmental Psychology*, 1972, **7**, 86.

Bieri, J. Parental identification, acceptability, authority, and within sex-differences in cognitive behavior. *Journal of Abnormal and Social Psychology*, 1960, **60**, 76–79.

Biller, H. B. Adults' conceptions of masculinity and femininity in children. Unpublished study, Emma Pendleton Bradley Hospital, Riverside, Rhode Island, 1966. (a)

Biller, H. B. Experiences with underachieving adolescents enrolled in an academic potential project. Unpublished manuscript, Emma Pendleton Bradley Hospital, Riverside, Rhode Island, 1966. (b)

Biller, H. B. A multiaspect investigation of masculine development in kindergarten age boys. *Genetic Psychology Monographs*, 1968, **76**, 89–139. (a)

Biller, H. B. A note on father-absence and masculine development in young lower class Negro and white boys. *Child Development*, 1968, **39**, 1003–1006. (b)

Biller, H. B. Father dominance and sex-role development in kindergarten age boys. *Developmental Psychology*, 1969, **1**, 87–94. (a)

Biller, H. B. Father-absence, maternal encouragement, and sex-role development in kindergarten age boys. *Child Development*, 1969, **40**, 539–546. (b)

Biller, H. B. Father-absence and the personality development of the male child. *Developmental Psychology*, 1970, **2**, 181–201.

Biller, H. B. *Father, child, and sex-role*. Lexington, Mass.: D. C. Heath, 1971. (a)

Biller, H. B. The mother-child relationship and the father-absent boy's personality development. *Merrill-Palmer Quarterly*, 1971, **17**, 227–241. (b)

Biller, H. B. Fathering and female sexual development. *Medical Aspects of Human Sexuality*, 1971, **5**, 116–138. (c)

Biller, H. B. Syndromes resulting from paternal deprivation in man. Paper presented at the Medical Research Council of Ireland's symposium on the Experimental Behavior Basis of Mental Disturbance, Galway, Ireland, April, 1972. (a)

Biller, H. B. Sex-role learning: Some comments and complexities from a multidimensional perspective. Paper presented at the Annual Meeting of the American Association for the Advancement of Science (Sec. 1). Symposium on Sex Role Learning in Childhood and Adolescence, Washington, D.C., December, 1972. (b)

Biller, H. B. *Paternal deprivation.* Lexington, Mass.: D. C. Heath, 1974, in press. (a)

Biller, H. B. Paternal and sex role factors in cognitive and academic functioning. In J. K. Cole & R. Dienstbier (Eds.), *Nebraska Symposium on Motivation.* Lincoln: University of Nebraska Press, 1974. Pp. 83–123. (b)

Biller, H. B., & Bahm, R. M. Father-absence, perceived maternal behavior, and masculinity of self-concept among junior high school boys. *Developmental Psychology,* 1971, **4**, 178–181.

Biller, H. B., & Barry, W. Sex role patterns, paternal similarity, and personality adjustment among college males. *Developmental Psychology,* 1971, **4**. 107.

Biller, H. B., & Borstelmann, L. J. Intellectual level and sex-role development in mentally retarded children. *American Journal of Mental Deficiency,* 1965, **70**, 443–447.

Biller, H. B., & Borstelmann, L. J. Masculine development: An integrative review. *Merril-Palmer Quarterly,* 1967, **13**, 253–294.

Biller, H. B., & Davids, A. Parent-child relations, personality development, and psychopathology. In A. Davids (Ed.), *Issues in abnormal child psychology.* Monterey, Calif.: Brooks/Cole, 1973. Pp. 48–77.

Biller, H. B., & Meredith, D. *Fathers and Children.* New York: David McKay, 1974, in press.

Biller, H. B., Singer, D. L., & Fullerton, M. Sex role development and creative potential in kindergarten age boys. *Developmental Psychology,* 1969, **1**, 291–296.

Biller, H. B., & Weiss, S. The father-daughter relationship and the personality development of the female. *Journal of Genetic Psychology,* 1970, **114**, 79–93.

Bing, E. Effect of child-rearing practices on development of differential cognitive abilities. *Child Development,* 1963, **34**, 631–648.

Blanchard, R. W., & Biller, H. B. Father-availability and academic performance among third grade boys. *Developmental Psychology,* 1971, **4**, 301–305.

Bronfenbrenner, U. Some familial antecedents of responsibility and leadership in adolescents. In L. Petrullo, & B. M. Bass (Eds.), *Leadership and interpersonal behavior.* New York: Holt, Rinehart & Winston, 1961. Pp. 239–272.

Bronfenbrenner, U. The psychological costs of quality and equality in education. *Child Development,* 1967, **38**, 909–925.

Brophy, J. E., & Laosa, L. M. The effect of a male teacher on the sex-typing of kindergarten children. *Proceedings of the 79th Annual Meeting of the American Psychological Association,* 1971, **6,** 169–170.

Burton, R. V., & Whiting, T. W. M. The absent father and cross-sex identity. *Merril-Palmer Quarterly,* 1961, **1,** 85–95.

Burton, R. V. Cross-sex identity in Barbados, *Developmental Psychology,* 1972, **6,** 365–374.

Busse, T. W. Child-rearing antecedents of flexible thinking. *Developmental Psychology,* 1969, **1,** 585–591.

Carlsmith, L. Effect of early father-absence on scholastic aptitude. *Harvard Educational Review,* 1969, **34,** 3–21.

Carter, E. S. How invalid are marks assigned by teachers? *Journal of Educational Psychology,* 1952, **43,** 218–228.

Cascario, E. F. The male teacher and reading achievement of first-grade boys and girls. Unpublished doctoral dissertation, Lehigh University, 1971.

Cervantes, L. F. Family background, primary relationships, and the high school dropout. *Journal of Marriage and the Family,* 1965, **27,** 218–223.

Chambers, J. A. Relating personality and biographical factors to scientific creativity. *Psychological Monographs,* 1964, **78,** (7), 584.

Coleman, J. S., Campbell, E. Q., McPartland, J., Mood, A. M., Weinfeld, R. D., & York, R. L. *Equality of educational opportunity.* Office of Education, 1966.

Corah, N. L. Differentiation in children and their parents. *Journal of Personality,* 1965, **33,** 300–308.

Cortés, D. F., & Fleming, E. The effects of father absence on the adjustment of culturally disadvantaged boys. *Journal of Special Education,* 1968, **2,** 413–420.

Crandall, V., Dewey, R., Katkovsky, W., & Preston, A. Parent's attitudes and behaviors and grade-school children's academic achievements. *Journal of Genetic Psychology,* 1964, **104,** 53–56.

Crescimbeni, J. Broken homes affect academic achievement. *Education,* 1964, **84,** 440–441.

Cross, H. J. The relation of parental training conditions to conceptual level in adolescent boys. *Journal of Personality,* 1966, **34,** 348–365.

Datta, L. E., & Parloff, M. B. Parent-child relationships and early scientific creativity. *Proceedings of the 75th Annual Convention of the American Psychological Association,* 1967, **2,** 149–150.

Dauw, D. C. Life experiences of original thinkers and good elaborators. *Exceptional Children,* 1966, **32,** 433–440.

Davids, A. *Abnormal children and youth.* New York: Wiley, 1972.

Davis, O., & Slobodian, J. Teacher behavior towards boys and girls in first grade reading instruction. *American Educational Research Journal,* 1967, **4,** 261–269.

Davis, A., & Havinghurst, R. J. Social class and color differences in child rearing. *American Sociological Review,* 1946, **11,** 698–710.

Deutsch, M. Minority group and class status as related to social and personality factors in scholastic achievement. *Monograph of the Society for Applied Anthropology,* 1960, **2,** 1–32.

Deutsch, M., & Brown, B. Social influences in Negro-white intelligence differences. *Journal of Social Issues,* 1964, **20,** 24–35.

Devereux, E. C., Jr., Bronfenbrenner, U., & Suci, G. J. Patterns of parent behavior in the United States and the Federal Republic of Germany: A cross-national comparison. *International Social Science Journal,* 1962, **14,** 488–506.

Downey, K. J. Parental interest in the institutionalized severely mentally retarded child. *Social Problems,* 1963, **11,** 186–193.

Dreyer, A., & Wells, M. Parental values, parental control, and creativity in young children. *Journal of Marriage and the Family,* 1966, **28,** 83–88.

Dyk, R. B., & Witkin, H. A. Family experiences related to the development of differentiation in children. *Child Development,* 1965, **36,** 21–55.

Dyl, A. S., & Biller, H. B. Paternal absence, social class, and reading achievement. Unpublished manuscript, University of Rhode Island, 1973.

Elder, G. H., Jr. *Adolescent achievement and mobility aspirations.* Chapel Hill, N.C.: Institute for Research in Social Science, 1962.

Engemoen, B. L. The influence of membership in a broken home on test performance of first grade children. Unpublished doctoral dissertation, North Texas University, 1966.

Epstein, R., & Liverant, S. Verbal conditioning and sex role identification in children. *Child Development,* 1963, **34,** 99–106.

Fagot, B. I., & Patterson, G. An in vivo analysis of reinforcing contingencies for sex-role behaviors in the pre-school child. *Developmental Psychology,* 1969, **1,** 563–568.

Farber, B. Effects of a severely mentally retarded child in the family. In E. P. Trapp & P. Himelstein (Eds.), *Readings on the exceptional child.* New York: Appleton-Century Crofts, 1962. Pp. 227–246.

Fish, K. D., & Biller, H. B. Perceived childhood paternal relationships and college females' personal adjustment. *Adolescence,* 1973, **8,** 415–420.

Garai, J. E., & Scheinfeld, A. Sex differences in mental and behavioral traits. *Genetic Psychology Monographs,* 1968, **77,** 169–299.

Gates, A. Sex differences in reading ability. *Elementary School Journal,* 1961, **61,** 431–434.

Grambs, J. D., & Waetjen, W. B. Being equally different: A new right for boys and girls. *National Elementary School Principal,* 1966, **46,** 59–67.

Gregory, I. Anterospective data following childhood loss of a parent: II. Pathology, performance, and potential among college students. *Archives of General Psychiatry,* 1965, **13,** 110–120.

Grunebaum, M. G., Hurwitz, I., Prentice, N. M., & Sperry, B. M. Fathers of sons with primary neurotic learning inhibition. *American Journal of Orthopsychiatry,* 1962, **32,** 462–473.

Hanson, E. H. Do boys get a square deal in school. *Education*, 1959, **79**, 597–598.

Hardy, M. C. Aspects of home environment in relation to behavior at the elementary school age. *Journal of Juvenile Research*, 1937, **21**, 206–225.

Heckscher, B. T. Household structure and achievement orientation in lower-class Barbadian families. *Journal of Marriage and the Family*, 1967, **29**, 521–526.

Heilbrun, A. B., Harrell, S. N., & Gillard, B. J. Perceived child rearing attitudes of fathers and cognitive control in daughters. *Journal of Genetic Psychology*, 1967, **111**, 29–40.

Helson, R. Personality characteristics and developmental history of creative college women. *Genetic Psychology Monographs*, 1967, **76**, 205–256.

Helson, R. Women mathematicians and the creative personality. *Journal of Consulting and Clinical Psychology*, 1971, **36**, 210–220.

Herzog, E., & Sudia, C. E. *Boys in fatherless families*. Washington: Office of Child Development, 1970.

Hetherington, E. M. A developmental study of the effects of sex of the dominant parent on sex-role preference, identification, and imitation in children. *Journal of Personality and Social Psychology*, 1965, **2**, 188–194.

Hetherington, E. M., Effects of paternal absence on sex-typed behaviors in Negro and white pre-adolescent males. *Journal of Personality and Social Psychology*, 1966, **4**, 87–91.

Hetherington, E. M. Effects of father absence on personality development in adolescent daughters. *Developmental Psychology*, 1972, **7**, 313–326.

Hilgard, J. R., Neuman, M. F., & Fisk, F. Strength of adults ego following bereavement. *American Journal of Orthopsychiatry*, 1960, **30**, 788–798.

Hoffman, M. L. Father absence and conscience development. *Developmental Psychology*, 1971, **4**, 400–406.

Holman, P. Some factors in the etiology of maladjustment in children. *Journal of Mental Science*, 1953, **99**, 654–688.

Honzik, M. P. Environmental correlates of mental growth: Prediction from the family setting at 21 months. *Child Development*, 1967, **38**, 338–364.

Hurley, J. R. Parental malevolence and children's intelligence. *Journal of Consulting Psychology*, 1967, **31**, 199–204.

Johnson, M. M. Sex-role learning in the nuclear family. *Child Development*, 1963, **34**, 319–333.

Kagan, J. Acquisition and significance of sex-typing and sex-role identity. In M. L. Hoffman & L. W. Hoffman (Eds.), *Review of child development research*. Vol. I, New York: Russell Sage, 1964. Pp. 137–167. (a)

Kagan, J. Sex typing during the preschool and early school years. In I. Janis, G. Mahl, J. Kagan, & R. Holt (Eds.), *Personality: Dynamics, development, and assessment*. New York: Harcourt, Brace & World, 1969.

Kelly, F. J., North, J., & Zingle, H. The relation of the broken homes to subsequent school behaviors. *Alberta Journal of Educational Research*, 1965, **11**, 215–219.

Kimball, B. The Sentence Completion Technique in a study of scholastic under-achievement. *Journal of Consulting Psychology*, 1952, **16**, 353–358.

Kohlberg, L. A cognitive-developmental analysis of children's sex-role concepts and attitudes. In E. E. Maccoby (Ed.) *The development of sex differences*. Stanford: Stanford University Press, 1966. Pp. 82–173.

Kohlberg, L., & Zigler, E. The impact of cognitive maturity on the development of sex-role attitudes in the years 4-8. *Genetic Psychology Monographs*, 1967, **75**, 89–165.

Katz, I. Socialization of academic motivation in minority group children. In D. Levine (Ed.), *Nebraska symposium on motivation*. Lincoln: University of Nebraska Press, 1967. Pp. 133–191.

Kohn, M. L. Social class and parental values. *American Journal of Sociology*, 1959, **64**, 337–351.

Kopel, D., & Geerded, H. A survey of clinical services for poor readers. *Journal of Educational Psychology Monograph*, 1933, **13**, 209–224.

Kyselka, W. Young men in nursery school. *Childhood Education*, 1966, **42**, 293–299.

Landy, F., Rosenberg, B. G., & Sutton-Smith, B. The effect of limited father-absence on cognitive development. *Child Development*, 1969, **40**, 941–944.

Lee, P. C., & Wolinsky, A. L. Male teachers of young children: A preliminary empirical study. *Young Children*, 1973, **28**, 342–352.

Lessing, E. E., Zagorin, S. W., & Nelson, D. WISC subtest and IQ score correlates of father absence. *Journal of Genetic Psychology*, 1970, **67**, 181–195.

Levy, D. M. *Maternal overprotection*. New York: Columbia University Press, 1943.

Lippitt, R., & Gold, M. Classroom social structure as a mental health problem. *Journal of Social Issues*, 1959, **15**, 40–58.

Long, B. H., Henderson, E. H., & Ziller, R. C. Self-social correlates of originality in children. *Journal of Genetic Psychology*, 1967, **111**, 47–54.

Lynn, D. B. *Parental and sex role identification*. Berkeley: McCutchan, 1969.

McClelland, D. C. *The achieving society*. Princeton, N.J.: Van Nostrand, 1961.

McCord, J., McCord, W., & Thurber, E. Some effects of paternal absence on male children. *Journal of Abnormal and Social Psychology*, 1962, **64**, 361–369.

McFarland, W. J. Are girls really smarter? *Elementary School Journal*, 1969, **70**, 14–19.

McNeil, J. D. Programmed instruction versus usual classroom procedures in teaching boys to read. *American Education Research Journal*, 1964, **1**, 113–119.

Maccoby, E. E. Sex differences in intellectual functioning. In E. E. Maccoby (Ed.), *The development of sex differences*. Stanford: Stanford University Press, 1966. Pp. 25–55.

Mackie, J. B., Maxwell, A. D., & Rafferty, F. T. Psychological development of culturally disadvantaged Negro kindergarten children: A study of the selective influence of family and school variables. Paper presented at the meeting of the American Orthopsychiatric Association, Washington, D.C., March, 1967.

Marzurkiewicz, A. J. Social-cultural influences and reading. *Journal of Developmental Reading,* 1960, **3**, 254–263.

Maslow, A. H. Creativity in self-actualizing people. In H. H. Anderson (Ed.), *Creativity and its cultivation.* New York: Harper, 1960.

Maxwell, A. E. Discrepancies between the pattern of abilities for normal and neurotic children. *Journal of Mental Science,* 1961, **107**, 300–307.

Medinnus, G. R. The relation between inter-parent agreement and several child measures. *Journal of Genetic Psychology,* 1965, **29**, 5–19.

Meyer, W., & Thompson, G. Sex differences in the distribution of teacher approval and disapproval among sixth grade children. *Journal of Educational Psychology,* 1956, **47**, 385–396.

Miller, W. B. Lower-class culture as a generating milieu of gang delinquency. *Journal of Social Issues,* 1958, **14**, 5–19.

Milton, G. A. The effects of sex-role identification upon problem solving skill. *Journal of Abnormal and Social Psychology,* 1957, **55**, 208–212.

Mischel, W. Father-absence and delay of gratification. *Journal of Abnormal and Social Psychology,* 1961, **62**, 116–124.

Mussen, P. H., Young, H. B., Godding, R., & Morante, L. The influence of father-son relationships on adolescent personality and attitudes. *Journal of Child Psychology and Psychiatry,* 1963, **4**, 3–16.

Mutimer, D., Loughlin, L., & Powell, M. Some differences in the family relationships of achieving and underachieving readers. *Journal of Genetic Psychology,* 1966, **109**, 67–74.

Nakamura, C. V., & Rogers, M. M. Parents' expectations of autonomous behavior and children's autonomy. *Developmental Psychology,* 1969, **1**, 613–617.

Nelsen, E. A., & Maccoby, E. E. The relationship between social development and differential abilities on the scholastic aptitude test. *Merill-Palmer Quarterly,* 1966, **12**, 269–289.

Ostrovsky, E. S. *Father to the child: Case studies of the experiences of a male teacher.* New York: Putnam, 1959.

Parker, S., & Kleiner, R. J. Characteristics of Negro mothers in single-headed households. *Journal of Marriage and the Family,* 1966, **28**, 507–513.

Pedersen, F. A. Relationships between father-absence and emotional disturbance in male military dependents. *Merrill-Palmer Quarterly,* 1966, **12**, 321–331.

Poffenberger, T. A., & Norton, D. Factors in the formation of attitudes toward mathematics. *Journal of Educational Research,* 1959, **52**, 171–176.

Plank, E. H., & Plank, R. Emotional components in arithmetic learning as seen through autobiographies. In R. S. Eissler et al. (Eds.), *The psychoanalytic study of the child.* Vol 9. New York: International Universities Press, 1954.

Polardy, J. N. What teachers believe, what children achieve. *Elementary School Journal,* 1969, **69**, 370–374.

Preston, R. Reading achievement of German and American children. *School and Society,* 1962, **90**, 350–354.

Radin, N. Father-child interaction and the intellectual functioning of four year old boys. *Developmental Psychology*, 1972, **6**, 353–361.

Radin, N. Observed paternal behaviors as antecedents of intellectual functioning in young boys. *Developmental Psychology*, 1973, **8**, 369–376.

Reuter, M. W., & Biller, H. B. Perceived paternal nurturance-availability and personality adjustment among college males. *Journal of Consulting and Clinical Psychology*, 1973, **40**, 339–342.

Risen, M. L. Relation of lack of one or both parents to school progress. *Elementary School Journal*, 1939, **39**, 528–531.

Rosen, B. C., and D'Andrade, R. The psychosocial origins of achievement motivation. *Sociometry*, 1959, **22**, 185–218.

Rouman, J. School children's problems as related to parental factors. *Journal of Educational Research*, 1956, **50**, 105–112.

Rowntree, G. Early childhood in broken families. *Population Studies*, 1955, **8**, 247–253.

Russell, I. L. Behavior problems of children from broken and intact homes. *Journal of Educational Sociology*, 1957, **31**, 125–129.

Ryans, D. G. *Characteristics of teachers*. Washington, D.C.: American Council on Education, 1960.

Santrock, J. W. Influence of onset and type of paternal absence on the first four Eriksonian developmental crises. *Developmental Psychology*, 1970, **3**, 273–274.

Santrock, J. W. Relation of type and onset of father-absence to cognitive development. *Child Development*, 1972, **43**, 455–469.

Seder, J. A. The origin of differences in extent of independence in children: Developmental factors in perceptual field dependence. Unpublished doctoral dissertation, Radcliffe College, 1957.

Sexton, P. C. *The feminized male: Classrooms, white collars, and the decline of manliness*. New York: Random House, 1969.

Siegman, A. W. Father-absence during childhood and antisocial behavior. *Journal of Abnormal Psychology*, 1966, **71**, 71–74.

Smelser, W. T. Adolescent and adult occupational choice as a function of family socioeconomic history. *Sociometry*, 1963, **4**, 393–409.

Solomon, D. The generality of children's achievement-related behavior. *Journal of Genetic Psychology*, 1969, **114**, 109–125.

Stein, A. H. The effects of sex-role standards for achievement and sex-role preference on three determinants of achievement motivation. *Developmental Psychology*, 1971, **4**, 219–231.

Stein, A. H., & Smithells, J. Age and sex differences in children's sex role standards about achievement. *Developmental Psychology*, 1969, **1**, 252–259.

Stein, A. H., Pohly, S. R., & Muellar, E. Sex-typing of achievement areas as a determinant of children's motivation and effort. Paper presented at the meeting of the Society for Research in Child Development, Santa Monica, California, March, 1969.

Stephens, W. N. *The Oedipus complex: Cross-cultural evidence.* Glencoe, Ill.; Free Press, 1962.

Strang, J. B. Students' reasons for becoming better readers. *Education,* 1968, **89,** 127–131.

Strodtbeck, F. L. Family interaction, values, and achievement. In D. C. McClelland et al. (Eds.), *Talent and society.* New York: Van Nostrand, 1958. Pp. 135–194.

Sutherland, H. E. G. The relationship between I.Q. and size of family in the case of fatherless children. *Journal of Genetic Psychology,* 1930, **38,** 161–170.

Sutton-Smith, B., Rosenberg, B. G., & Landy F. Father-absence effects in families of different sibling compositions. *Child Development,* 1968, **38,** 1213–1221.

Tallman, I. Spousal role differentiation and the socialization of severely retarded children. *Journal of Marriage and the Family,* 1965, **27,** 37–42.

Terman, L. M., & Oden, M. H. *The gifted child grows up.* Stanford: Stanford University Press, 1947.

Thomes, M. M. Children with absent fathers. *Journal of Marriage and the Family,* 1968, **30,** 89–96.

Triplett, L. Elementary education—a man's world? *The Instructor,* 1968, **78,** 50–52.

Van der Veen, F. The parent's concept of the family unit and child adjustment. *Journal of Counseling Psychology,* 1965, **12,** 196–200.

Veroff, J., Atkinson, J., Feld, S., & Gurin, G. The use of thematic apperception to assess motivation in a nationwide interview study. *Psychological Monographs,* 1960, **74,** (Whole No. 499).

Weisberg, P. S. & Springer, K. J. Environment factors in creative function: a study of gifted children. *Archives of General Psychiatry,* 1961, **5,** 554–564.

Witkin, H. A. The problem of individuality in development. In B. Kaplan & S. Wapner (Eds.), *Perspectives in psychological theory.* New York: International Universities Press, 1960. Pp. 335–361.

Witkin, H. A., Dyk, R. B., Faterson, H., Goodenough, D. R., & Karp, S. A. *Psychological differentation: Studies of development.* New York: Wiley, 1962.

Wohlford, P., & Liberman, D. Effect of father absence on personal time, field independence, and anxiety. *Proceedings of the 78th Annual Convention of The American Psychological Association,* 1970, **5,** 263–264.

Wyer, R. S. Self-acceptance, discrepancy between parents' perceptions of their children, and goal-seeking effectiveness. *Journal of Personality and Social Psychology,* 1965, **2,** 311–316.

CHAPTER 2

Relation of Learning in Childhood
to Psychopathology and Aggression
in Young Adulthood

LEONARD D. ERON, MONROE M. LEFKOWITZ, LEOPOLD O. WALDER,
AND L. ROWELL HUESMANN

Aggression, when it refers to harmful behavior directed against living organisms or property, is usually considered to be maladaptive behavior not unlike other expressions of psychopathology. Thus it would seem that the learning conditions which precede the appearance of aggressive behavior should be similar to the antecedents of other types of maladaptive behavior.

The focus of this chapter is on the relations that exist between learning conditions present in the environment of boys and girls when they are eight years old and the maladaptive behaviors they exhibit 10 years later. Both aggression and a more general expression of psychopathology are considered, and the impact of differential socializing experiences of boys and girls is treated.

Interest in the effect of learning conditions on the development of maladaptive forms of behavior stems largely from the experience of clinicians who over the years have observed that their patients' childhood histories often contain evidence of unusual disciplinary practices utilized by their patients' parents. Learning theory, psychoanalysis, and other developmental theories of personality also emphasize the importance of early experience on later behavior. However, approximately 10 years ago, when Frank (1965) reviewed research over a 40-year period on the role of the family in the development of personality and psychopathology, he was forced to conclude that there was no consistent evidence on the link between parent–child relations in early childhood and the development of psychopathology. This was not unlike the earlier conclusion of Orlansky (1949) that there was no consistent support for the presence of a relation between personality development and such infant experiences as feeding, toilet training, and thumb sucking.

In 1960, however, we completed a study that demonstrated a positive relation between certain parental disciplinary practices in middle childhood and aggressive behavior exhibited concurrently by children in school. Ten years later in a follow-up study done on a large sample of the original population it was demonstrated:

1. That it is possible to predict from indications of aggressive behavior in middle childhood to later behavior.
2. That certain parental practices persisted in their relation to aggressive behavior 10 years later while other practices seemed to lose their effect.
3. That the causal direction of the relation seemed to go from learning conditions to aggressive behavior.
4. That aggressive behavior was related to other indications of psychopathology.
5. That, while some parental practices were propaedeutic to aggression, others were more apt to lead to different manifestations of behavior disturbance.

The original focus of the longitudinal study to be described in this chapter was on mental health. Because of the many difficulties inherent in doing objective studies of such a loosely defined general concept, we chose aggression as one aspect of mental health which was possible to define, observe, and measure. Aggression was defined as "an act which injures or irritates another person [Walder, Abelson, Eron, Banta, & Laulicht, 1961]." This signifies hostile, interpersonal aggression without any implication of intent. It does not refer to the more positive connotations of the term that imply striving and achievement motivation although, as will become apparent, the two aspects of aggression are not unrelated.

LONGITUDINAL STUDY—FIRST WAVE

The first wave of the study, conducted in 1960, entailed the classroom testing of the entire population of third graders in a semirural county in the Hudson River Valley of New York, and individual interviews with their mothers and fathers.

A peer nomination measure consisting of 10 items of aggressive behavior constituted the measure of aggression in the third grade. Sample items were: "Who pushes or shoves children?" "Who says mean things?" "Who takes other children's things without asking?" The reliability and validity of this measure have been demonstrated in numerous studies (Eron, Walder, & Lefkowitz, 1971; Walder et al., 1961). Measures of the learning conditions were taken from parent interviews conducted individually in face-to-face situations. These interviews, completely objective and precoded, yielded measures on four general types of variables presumed to be antecedent to aggression in children—instigators, reinforcers, identification, and social class. These were hypothesized to be the learning conditions of aggression. Instigation referred to conditions in the home which would likely be frustrating to the child and thus spark aggressive behavior. Reinforcement referred to contingent response by the parent to the child's aggression. Identification had two aspects—internalization of parental standards and modeling of behavior after significant adults. These could either inhibit or facilitate aggressive behavior. Social class variables were included, since they are hypothesized to affect development of personality in a variety of ways.

The data obtained from the 875 subjects when they were in the third grade and that from their mothers and fathers have been analyzed, and the results reported extensively elsewhere (Eron et al., 1971). It is fair to say that all the major findings are consistent with the hypothesis that aggression may be learned by a child from his interaction with the environment. Each of the four classes of variables presumed to be the learning conditions of aggression related both independently and in interaction to aggression observed in school. Generally, the less nurturant and accepting the parents were toward the child at home, the more aggressive he was in school; the more the child was punished for aggression at home, the more aggressive he was in school; and the less identified the child was with either or both parents, the more aggressive he was in school. One of the major instigators to aggression in children seemed to be a general lack of favorable support from both parents which in turn tended to reduce the effectiveness of any punishment the parent administered as a deterrent to aggressive behavior. Furthermore, parental punitiveness, especially physical punishment, may have provided a model of aggressive behavior for the child to emulate. Other models of aggression were furnished on the children's favorite TV programs.

The difficulty with such a one-time field study is that causation cannot be teased apart from correlation. In the example above, was punishment correlated with aggression because an aggressive child is punished more or because many children imitate the punishments they receive, or both? To separate causation and correlation, one needs to obtain repeated measurements on a child during his development. With such longitudinal data one can perhaps go beyond correlational theories and distinguish between the plausibility of rival causal theories.

LONGITUDINAL STUDY—FOLLOW-UP WAVE

Thus in 1970, 10 years after the original data collection period, we attempted to reinterview our original third-grade population, then about 19 years old, to see if the behaviors learned in the earlier period persisted into the later one, and if the learning conditions that were delineated 10 years earlier still demonstrated their effects (Lefkowitz, Eron, Walder, & Huesmann, 1971).

Subjects

We were successful in obtaining complete interviews from 427 subjects in the second time period, referred to hereafter as the 13th grade. These subjects included 211 boys and 216 girls. Modal age was 19 and on the average they had completed 12.6 years of schooling (in addition to kindergarten). Based on the 25% for whom current IQ scores could be obtained, the mean 12th grade IQ was 109.1 ± 11.6. As judged by father's occupation they were predominantly a middle-class group (Warner, Meeker, & Eells, 1960), probably not too different from what one would find in similar localities across the country.

On the other hand, the 427 subjects who were reinterviewed were not a completely representative sample of the original 875 in the third grade. In particular, the 13th-grade sample included more of the original low-aggression subjects and less of the original high-aggression subjects than one would have expected by chance. Of the boys in the lower quartile of aggression in the third grade, 57% were reinterviewed. However, of the boys who had been in the upper quartile in the third grade, only 27% were reinterviewed. The corresponding figures for girls were 63 and 33%. Why would almost double the number of low aggressive subjects as compared to high aggressive subjects appear for the reinterview 10 years later? The most compelling single explanation we can offer is based on a relation we discovered between a family's residential mobility and its child's aggressiveness. We found these factors to be positively correlated within our reinterview sample $(r = .17, p < .05$, for boys); thus it is likely that the families of high-aggressive children were more likely to have moved between the times of the two interviews than the families of low aggressive subjects. One explanation might be that residential mobility serves as a frustration by providing the child new situations he must adjust to in the neighborhood and at school.

Criterion Measures

During the interview, lasting about 2 hours, we obtained information about the subjects' current status, behavior, and attitudes, and had the subjects again rate their peers on aggressive behaviors. One of the most obvious findings in the longitudinal study was the stability of aggressive behavior over a 10-year period for both boys and girls (see Table 1). This was something more than reliability of ratings. Aside from the fact that there was a 10-year lag making it highly unlikely that memory of earlier ratings was an important factor, each subject was rated by a somewhat different set of raters in the later period. Originally there had been 38 different third-grade classes in which children were rated only by members of their third-grade classroom. These 38 classes fed into five different high schools. In the follow-up interview each subject was presented with the third-grade lists of all the feeder classes for the high school he attended in addition to his own third-grade class, and was asked to indicate all those students he knew and could rate. This then was the group of subjects any particular subject rated.

Thus there were two different groups of raters—overlapping, but different. In the third grade each child performed this peer-nomination task in a classroom setting while in the 13th grade it was in a face-to-face interview. In either case a child's raw aggression rating was computed by adding up the number of times he was named by his peers on the aggression items and dividing by the total number of questions. In the third grade there were 10 items but in the 13th grade only nine because one third-grade item was judged to be inappropriate for 19-year-old subjects. To correct for the fact that a well-known subject might be named more often than another subject even though both were equally aggressive, a subject's raw aggression rating was divided by an estimate of the number of people who could have named him. In the third grade this was the number of children present in the classroom on the day of the testing; but in the 13th grade one could name any subject; so a subject's raw aggression score was divided by the number of times he was nominated by all others on the question, which was asked of each respondent, "Who do you know?".

Since most of the subjects had now been out of high school for a year and were probably not in current contact with their peers, the questions had to be phrased in the past tense. This suggests the possibility that 13th-grade ratings might simply be a remeasure of 3rd-grade aggression ratings; however, the available evidence argues strongly against this interpretation. First, only those subjects who reappeared for the interview were used as raters in the 13th grade. It seems likely that most of them had known each other in recent years. Second, as part of the instructions, subjects were told, "base your answers on what you *last* knew of each person from personal observation and contact." Finally, and most importantly, the 13th-grade peer ratings closely agree with the other 13th-grade measures of aggression to be discussed below, but the third-grade peer ratings do not correlate well with these other 13th-grade measures. Of course, the nominations made in the 13th grade were undoubtedly influenced to some extent by behaviors prior to the 13th grade, but the resulting 13th-grade aggression scores are clearly measures of more recent behaviors than were the third-grade scores.

During the reinterview in the 13th grade each subject was tested with the MMPI (Hathaway & McKinley, 1969). It has been reported that elevations on scale 4 and 9 of this test are indicative of delinquency (Hathaway & Monarchesi, 1961). Hence we added together each subject's T-scores on scales 4 and 9

Table 1.   Correlations Between Peer-Ratings and Self-Ratings of Aggression

	Peer-Rating, Age 8	Peer-Rating, Age 19	Self-Rating, Age 19	MMPI 4&9, Age 19
Peer-rating, age 8		$.38^c$	$.16^a$	$.21^b$
Peer-rating, age 19	$.47^c$		$.50^c$	$.39^c$
Self-rating, age 19	$.07$	$.24^b$		$.46^c$
MMPI 4&9, age 19	$.13^a$	$.28^b$	$.45^c$	

Boys' correlations above diagonal.
Girls' correlations below diagonal.
^{a}p < .05.
^{b}p < .01.
^{c}p < .001.

of the MMPI to get a score reflecting potential antisocial behavior. This measure correlated positively with 13th-grade peer-rated aggression (see Table 1). The MMPI psychotic tetrad score (see discussion of psychopathology below) was also used as a measure of psychopathology.

To secure self-reports of aggression from our subjects in the 13th grade, we included two sets of questions in the interview. One set was designed to have face validity as a measure of a subject's propensity for antisocial behavior, and the other set was designed to measure the intensity of a subject's aggressive habits. In the former set there were 26 questions such as; "In the last three years, how many times have you taken something from a store without paying for it?" "How many times in the last three years have you hit someone badly enough to need bandages or a doctor?"

In the latter set there were rating scales on which the subject checked one of the following: almost always true; often true; sometimes true; seldom true; never true; which best expressed his acceptance of items like: "I feel like swearing," "I feel like being a little rude to people," "I feel like picking a fight or arguing with people." The questions in both these sets had been derived through extensive pretesting. A Total Aggressive Habit score was obtained by summing the scores on all the questions from both sets. This self-rating score correlated highly with 13th-grade peer-rated aggression (see Table 1).

Each of the measures above of aggression possesses reasonable face validity. In addition, their demonstrated statistical interrelatedness supports their validity. With regard to reliability, however, we only have information on the MMPI and peer-rating measures, both of which are highly reliable (Eron et al., 1971; Hathaway & McKinley, 1969).

Do these aggression variables measure the type of aggression in which we are interested— "an act which injures or irritates another person?" To try to answer this question, we asked the New York State Division of Criminal Justice, which collects data on arrests within the state, to determine the number of arrests of male subjects who were low and high on aggression in the third grade. The results indicated that three times as many subjects who were in the high quartile as were in the low were mentioned as having been arrested sometime before age 20. Because the total number of arrests was small the data are only suggestive but they tend to support the contention that our aggression measures are valid and the consistency in peer-rating over a 10-year period indicates that aggressive behavior is stable over time and predictive from grade three to a year beyond high school (i.e., age eight to 19).

It is interesting that we were able to get such high correlations between self- and peer-ratings in the 13th grade although there had been no such correlation in the third grade. Perhaps at age 19 subjects can describe themselves better; or they feel it is less incriminating to admit these behaviors to an interviewer who is a stranger and whom they will probably never see again than when they were in a classroom in grade three and had no real assurance that the teacher would not see their answers. Or perhaps it might even be the difference in the times—in 1960, it was not the "in thing" for young people to engage in or admit to certain antisocial behaviors which now are acceptable at least to persons in this age group. "Ripping off" is the term currently used to legitimize stealing and make it socially acceptable. In 1960, there was no such term.

Having established the credibility of these as measures of aggression we may now turn our attention to what the relation is of the parent–child rearing variables measured when the child was eight years old to his or her aggressive behavior at age 19. As stated previously, we were predicting from four classes of antecedent variables: instigators, contingent responses, identification, and social class. This information was obtained primarily from parent interviews, but there were also classroom procedures with the third-grade children which measured variables considered to be antecedents.

Antecedent Measures

Instigators

An instigator to a behavior is a stimulus that usually elicits the behavior in question as a response. In third-grade subjects we measured four major characteristics of our subjects and their families which we considered potential instigators of aggression: *parental rejection of the child; parental disharmony; lack of nurturance of the child by the parents; and the child's IQ*. This last variable, measured with the California Test of Mental Maturity (Sullivan, Clark, & Tiegs, 1957), was obtained as a control measure, but upon reflection we hypothesized that low IQ might act as a frustrator and thus be an instigator to aggression. The other three instigation variables were scored from interviews with the parents. The questions employed were selected and validated with procedures described elsewhere (Eron et al., 1971). A very high score on the rejection scale would represent a parent who complains that his child is too forgetful, has bad manners, does not read as well as he should, does not take care of his things, does not follow directions, wastes too much time, and has poor taste in what he buys for himself. A high score on the disharmony scale would represent parents who disagreed with each other about their choice of friends and social life, who spend little of their time together, who can think of nothing they like to do together, who have serious arguments in front of the children about how to raise them, who have left home during arguments, and who are disinterested in each other's work. Finally, a very low score on nurturance would be achieved by a parent who does not know why his child cries, what upsets his child, or what his child fears; who does not have time to talk to his child; and who cannot say how he shows his child that "he is on his side."

Contingent Responses to Aggression

While instigators may trigger aggressive acts, the development of more enduring aggressive habits should be influenced by how a subject's environment responds to his aggressiveness. Among the most important reinforcing agents for an eight-year-old or younger child are undoubtedly his parents; so in the third grade we selected the parents' use of punishment as a measure of how a child's aggressive acts are reinforced. An assumption underlying this choice was that those parents who employ less punishment resort to positive reinforcement to control the child's behavior. However, looking back, we see that it was a mistake not to assess the extent of positive reinforcement of nonaggressive behaviors on the part of the child by the parent. In any case punishment scores were computed separately for each parent and averaged to obtain an overall score. The higher the score, the more punishment a parent said he used in controlling his child.

Identification

The importance of modeling and observational learning in the acquisition of behavior has become increasingly clear in recent years. The child does what he sees being done especially if he sees that behavior being reinforced (Bandura & Walters, 1963; Bandura, Ross, & Ross, 1963b). While various characteristics of the model and the situation influence the likelihood of immediate imitation (Bandura, 1969), observational learning would seem to have great potential as a determiner of life long patterns of behavior.

A second type of identification relevant to the development of personality is the psychoanalytic concept of internalization of parents' values, desires, and standards (Freud, 1923). The child who successfully internalizes his parents' standards finds it easy to control his own behavior in line with his parents' proscriptions.

Identification by Modeling. Both types of identification variables, modeling, and internalization were measured in the third grade. The modeling category included the child's copying of parental behaviors, his sex-role modeling, and his potential for modeling aggressive behaviors observed on television. To measure the *child's identification with each parent,* we calculated an "Expressive Behavior Profile" for both parents and for the child. In this procedure, a variation of the *Semantic Differential Technique* (Osgood, Suci, & Tannenbaum, 1957), the subject rated several of his own expressive behaviors, for example, walking and talking, on 18 five-point scales with bipolar adjectives as anchors, for example, fast-slow. Since parents were also asked to rate themselves on the behaviors, a measure of discrepancy between the child and each of his parents could be obtained. The total discrepancy between a parent and child was the square root of the sum of the squared discrepancies on each bipolar adjective scale.

The child's *sex-role identification* was measured by the Games and Activities Preference List (Lefkowitz, 1962). Each third-grade child was presented with a list of questions requiring him or her to choose between two activities. For example: "Would you rather go shooting or go bowling?" "Would you rather use lipstick and powder or use a razor and shaving cream?" The hypothesis which led to the development and use of this measure of identification was that preference for masculine activities would be positively related to aggression (Lefkowitz, 1962).

Television Violence. With the increasing prominence of violence in our society, television, with its heavy emphasis on interpersonal violence and acquisitive lawlessness, is proposed as a model that teaches the child aggressive habits. The effect on aggressive behavior of viewing aggressive visual displays has been demonstrated in the laboratory in many experiments with children (Bandura, Ross, & Ross, 1963a). With this longitudinal field study we hoped to test the effects of a steady exposure to violent television models upon the development of a child's aggressiveness.

The child's exposure to aggressive models on television was measured in the third grade by asking the mother to name the child's three favorite television programs. All programs mentioned were then categorized as violent or nonviolent by two independent raters with 94% agreement in their ratings. Differences in the remaining 6% of the programs were resolved by mutual discussion between the raters. Each subject received a score according to the number of violent television programs he was reported by his mother as favoring. Scores ranged from 1 (for no violent programs) to 4 (for three violent programs).

Ten years later each subject himself was asked for his four current favorite television programs. Again all programs were categorized for presence or absence of violence by two independent raters who were only a few years older than the subjects. Scores, assigned to each program on the basis of agreement between the raters, ranged from 0 when both raters said nonviolent, to 1 when they disagreed, to 2 when both said violent. Here again there was good agreement between the two raters. They agreed on 81% of 125 programs mentioned by the subjects. The score given a subject was the sum of the violence ratings for the four programs he mentioned.

The designation by these raters of violent and nonviolent programs agreed very well with the assignment of programs by Feshbach and Singer (1971) to aggressive and nonaggressive diets in their field experiment. Furthermore, the judgments of our raters were in close agreement with the results obtained by Greenberg and Gordon (1970), who did an extensive rating study in which they used as raters both established TV critics and 300 persons randomly selected from the telephone directory. We recomputed our subjects' 13th-grade television violence scores on the basis of the Greenberg and Gordon rating and found a .94 correlation between the resulting scores and ours.

Three other aspects of the subjects' television viewing habits were assayed in this study. We had the mothers (in the third grade) and the subjects themselves (in the 13th grade) estimate how many *hours of television the subject watched* each week. In addition, we had the subjects report in the 13th grade on their *sports viewing habits* and their feelings about *how realistic television* seems to be.

Identification by Internalization. Identification with parents through internalization of values was assessed by the amount of *confessing* to his parents that the child performed and the amount of *guilt* the child expressed to his parents. Both of these behaviors were reported by each parent when the subjects were eight years old. A child low on confessing would be one who, according to his parents, always denies doing "naughty" acts. A child low on guilt would be one who, according to his parents, feels that his punishments are not justified, doesn't worry about lies, tries to get away with things he shouldn't when he thinks no one is watching, and who does not feel sorry when he disobeys.

Sociocultural Variables

Sociocultural variables can be hypothesized to affect the development of personality in a variety of ways ranging from genetic predispositions, to nutrition, to learning. In choosing the variables to represent a subject's sociocultural environment, we entertained no particular hypotheses about the processes underlying their effect; rather we tried to be exhaustive in our coverage of potential sociocultural predictors of aggression. In both the third and 13th grades we rated the *status of the father's occupation* on a seven-point scale with low numbers representing high status (Warner et al., 1960). Besides occupational status we evaluated the parents' general *mobility orientation*. A parent high on *mobility orientation* would be very willing to learn new skills, leave his friends, move, take on more responsibility, and give up spare time to get ahead. The *ethnic background* of the family was also assessed. A highly ethnic family would be one in which one parent or all the grandparents were born in another country. Finally, both the *religious background* of the family and the *frequency of church attendance* as reported by the parents were recorded as well as the parents' education.

RESULTS AND DISCUSSION—AGGRESSION

The basic multivariate analyses upon which our conclusions are based are multiple regression equations computed to predict both synchronous and later aggression from the independent variables. In a multiple regression analysis a coefficient is computed for each independent (predictor) variable so that the weighted sum of the independent variables yields the best possible prediction of the value of the dependent variable. As Darlington (1968) and others have pointed out, one can treat the standardized coefficients in a multiple regression equation as measures of the relative contributions of the independent variables in determining the dependent variable.

The multiple regressions were computed in a stepwise manner with only those independent variables being entered that could account for at least 2% of the variance in the criterion aggression variable. The regressions for 128 boys are shown in Table 2 while the regressions for 120 girls are shown in Table 3.*

We did separate analyses for boys and girls because preliminary analysis indicated that the measures of aggression distinguished the males from the females. There were statistically significant differences between males' and females' mean scores on every measure of aggression in both grades. The differences were more pronounced in the 13th grade. In addition, a principal component factor analysis of subjects' sex and the variables that were used in the study yielded a first principal factor whose largest loading was for the subjects' sex and whose next largest loadings were for the measures of aggression. Finally, a comparison of girls in the highest quartile of aggression with those in the lowest quartile revealed a difference in profiles on the MMPI: The high-aggressive girls were significantly more masculine in their interests and attitudes. Because of these findings the data for males and females were analyzed separately.

In addition to the multivariate analyses, Pearsonian correlations were computed between each of the third-grade predictor variables and the aggression cri-

---

*These multiple regression equations differ slightly from comparable regression equations published previously (Eron, Huesmann, Lefkowitz, & Walder, 1972) for two reasons. First, certain additional independent variables were considered in the present analysis. Second, only those subjects for whom data on every independent variable were available entered into the current analyses.

Table 2. Multiple Regression Analyses for Boys [a]

Third-Grade Predictor Variable	Type	Predicting Third-Grade Aggression		Predicting 13th-Grade Aggression	
		Standardized Coefficient	Significance	Standardized Coefficient	Significance
Parental rejection of child	Instigator	.248	$p < .004$		
Parental disharmony	Instigator				
Child's IQ	Instigator	-.230	$p < .005$		
Parental nurturance of child	Instigator	-.305	$p < .001$	-.166	$p < .041$
Parental punishment of child	Contingent				
Child's identification with father	Identification				
Father's aggressiveness	Identification				
Child's identification with mother	Identification			-.191	$p < .020$
Mother's aggressiveness	Identification				
TV violence	Identification	.166	$p < .038$	.251	$p < .003$
Child's guilt	Identification				
Child's confessing to parents	Identification				
Child's preference for boys' games	Identification				
Child's preference for girls' games	Identification	-.141	$p < .075$	-.189	$p < .023$
Father's occupational status	Socio-cultural	-.203	$p < .011$		
Parents' mobility orientation	Socio-cultural			.271	$p < .002$
Parents' religiosity (frequency of church attendance)	Socio-cultural				
Parents' educational level	Socio-cultural				
Ethnicity of family	Socio-cultural			-.137	$p < .095$
		$R = .535, p < .001$		$R = .499, p < .001$	

[a] The regressions were computed in a stepwise manner. Stepping was stopped when no variable could be entered which would explain at least 2% of the variance in the criterion aggression variable.

Table 3. Multiple Regression Analyses for Girls [a]

Third-Grade Predictor Variable	Type	Predicting Third Grade Aggression		Predicting 13th-Grade Aggression	
		Standardized Coefficient	Significance	Standardized Coefficient	Significance
Parental rejection of child	Instigator	.322	$p < .001$		
Parental disharmony	Instigator				
Child's IQ	Instigator			-.119	$p < .186$
Parental nurturance of child	Instigator				
Parental punishment of child	Contingent				
Child's identification with father	Identification			-.175	$p < .05$
Father's aggressiveness	Identification				
Child's identification with mother	Identification	-.289	$p < .001$		
Mother's aggressiveness	Identification				
TV violence	Identification			-.172	$p < .04$
Child's guilt	Identification			-.143	$p < .100$
Child's confessing to parents	Identification	-.202	$p < .012$		
Child's preference for boys' games	Identification				
Child's preference for girls' games	Identification				
Father's occupational status	Socio-cultural	-.293	$p < .002$	-.332	$p < .001$
Parents' mobility orientation	Socio-cultural			.172	$p < .044$
Parents' religiosity (frequency of church attendance)	Socio-cultural			-.192	$p < .025$
Parents' educational level	Socio-cultural	.152	$p < .103$	.261	$p < .015$
Ethnicity of family	Socio-cultural	.165	$p < .033$		
		$R = .602, p < .001$		$R = .534, p < .001$	

[a] The regressions were computed in a stepwise manner. Stepping was stopped when no variable could be entered which would explain at least 2% of the variance in the criterion aggression variable.

Table 4. Correlations Between Third-Grade Predictor Variables And Aggression In The Third And 13th Grades

Third-Grade Predictor Variables	Aggression			
	Third Grade		Thirteenth Grade	
	Boys	Girls	Boys	Girls
Parental rejection of child	$.28^b$	$.35^c$	.10	.04
Preental disharmony	$-.08$	$.17^a$	.07	.12
Parental nurturance of child	$-.16$	$-.02$	$-.15$	$-.09$
Child's IQ	$-.29^b$	$-.28^b$	$-.18^b$	$-.19^b$
Parental punishment of child	$.18^a$	.12	.13	.04
Child's identification with father	$-.25^b$	$-.22^a$	$-.16^a$	$-.22^a$
Father's aggressiveness	.01	.02	.11	.06
Child's identification with mother	$-.23^b$	$-.30^b$	$-.17^a$	$-.19^a$
Mother's aggressiveness	.01	.12	.03	.06
TV violence	$.21^b$	$-.02$	$.31^b$	$-.13$
Child's guilt	$-.14$	$-.34^c$	$-.05$	$-.20^a$
Child's confessing to parent	$-.19^b$	$-.31^b$	$-.18^b$	$-.14$
Child's preference for boys' games	.11	.04	.11	.02
Child's preference for girls' games	$-.16^a$	$-.04$	$-.17^a$	$-.01$
Father's occupational status	$-.16^a$	$-.16^a$	.03	$-.14$
Parents' mobility orientation	.15	.02	$.25^b$	.06
Parents' frequency of church attendance	.04	$-.18^a$	.09	$-.20^a$
Parents' educational level	$-.05$	.06	.07	.13
Ethnicity of family	$-.13$	.07	$-.07$	.08

$^a p < .05.$
$^b p < .01.$
$^c p < .001.$

teria at the third and 13th grades. These data are presented for both boys and girls in Table 4.*

The overall theme suggested by these analyses and which forms the basis for the remainder of this paper is the following: while the occurrence of the instigators to aggression is a good predictor of a child's immediate or synchronous aggression, the best predictors of aggression longitudinally are the identification variables and sociocultural variables.

Let us now consider the implications of the regression analyses and other associated bivariate analyses for each of the four classes of independent variables: instigators to aggression; contingent responses to aggression; identification; and sociocultural variables.

---

*The correlation coefficients were computed using the largest number of subjects available. Thus in some cases the N's are greater than those in the multivariate analyses.

Instigators

Within the class of variables termed instigators, rejection was the most prominent predictor of synchronous aggression, predicting well for both boys and girls. Also, low nurturance and low IQ were strong predictors of synchronous aggression for boys. Although low IQ for girls and lack of nurturance for boys predict aggression longitudinally, the predictive power of IQ and nurturance are greatly reduced. It seems fair to say that in a multivariate context none of the instigator variables predicts very well to later aggression. Instigators are perhaps necessary antecedents to comtemporaneous aggression, but apparently their effect is short-lived and other variables are more important in predicting later aggression.

IQ was included in the class of instigators on the hypothesis that the frustrations of coping with a low IQ would lead to higher aggression. In fact low IQ was consistently correlated with high aggression for both boys and girls within our sample as illustrated in Tables 2, 3, and 4. Another interpretation of low IQ is not as an instigator but rather as a condition which limits a child's ability to learn a variety of socially acceptable behaviors. Such a child's repertory of behavior may be constricted in comparison with that of a child of average or high IQ. The low IQ child simply has more difficulty learning to behave in a nonaggressive manner. Such a child finds it easier to learn the direct and salient behaviors. The child with a higher IQ has more learning options open to him so that he is able to learn a wider variety of social behaviors.

Perhaps a better measure of instigation to aggression associated with low IQ is school achievement. In support of this observation we found a $-.39$ correlation $(p < .01)$ between achievement test scores in high school and synchronous aggression for girls and $-.36$ $(p < .01)$ for boys. Indeed Semler and Eron (1967) found that among third-grade boys achievement explained the major portion of the variance in the relation between IQ scores and aggression.

Contingent Responses to Aggression

Contingent response to aggression, which, when studied in the third grade with a much larger sample (Eron et al., 1963), seemed to be a very important variable in determining aggressive behavior of boys at that time, does not seem so important when examined in the longitudinal context of the multiple regression analysis. With the attenuated sample (only those who were reinterviewed) punishment does not serve as a predictor to aggression. However, the bivariate correlation as seen in Table 4 is significant in the third grade and approaches significance in the 13th grade. Furthermore, when the subjects are partitioned into groups having high, medium, and low punishing parents, an interesting pattern of relations among mean scores emerges which the correlation coefficient may actually be masking (Table 5). This is likely to happen when the variables are skewed or nonlinear effects otherwise exist. It is seen from this table that the

Table 5.   Mean Aggression Scores of Boys at Age 19 According to Punishment by Parents at Age Eight

	Aggression Scores	
Punishment	Unadjusted	Adjusted[a]
Low	87.4	89.4
Medium	67.4	66.5
High	89.2	88.1

[a]These scores have been adjusted for covariation with aggression score in the third grade.

least aggressive boys are those whose parents are moderately punitive toward aggressive behavior. When parents are either very permissive or harshly punitive toward aggression by their sons, these boys in late adolescence tend to be more aggressive. It should be emphasized this is not a statistically significant effect but only a suggestive trend.

It will be recalled that at age eight there were opposite findings for highly identified and moderately identified boys in regard to punishment by father. The analysis was repeated in the 13th grade with the attenuated sample. The previous results were not replicated, indicating that the moderating influence of identification on the effect of punishment does not persist until age 19.

Identification

As can be seen from the regression analyses and the bivariate correlations, the identification variables are much more successful in predicting aggression both synchronously and longitudinally. Two of the identification measures, children's confessing and guilt as reported by parents, are often viewed as indications of the child's internalization of parental interdictions, and, when viewed in a dynamic model of behavior, are indications of conscience that develop through identification with parents.

It is instructive to consider the child behaviors which are associated with high amounts of confessing and of guilt. These behaviors are a form of communication from the child—a self-disclosure about some negative or undesirable action on his or her part. The fact that a child admits a transgression to a parent suggests that the parent has supported such communications and is probably a positively reinforcing agent for the child. If so, a child with high scores on our measures of identification might well have a parent who uses a child management system which includes positive aspects. Such systems are much more effective in building behavior controls which are mediated by the child himself and are not as situationally or time bound as predominantly negative control systems. This might explain why identification variables are effective across time and why externally imposed conditions such as punishment are not. It has been demonstrated (Azrin, 1958; Chasdi & Lawrence, 1955) that punishment has an effect only when the punishing agent is likely to be there; while positive reinforcement has a more pervasive effect on behavior.

In confirmation of our hypothesis concerning identification and aggression, identification as measured by confessing behavior was negatively correlated with aggression for both boys and girls at both time periods. The measure of guilt behaves in the same fashion in its negative relationship to aggressive behavior but less consistently, especially for boys. For girls the regression equations show that confessing behavior is a predictor of low aggression synchronously, while guilt behavior predicts low aggression later in life. Perhaps the most consistent relationships between identification and aggression occurred as a function of a child's identification with his parents in expressive behavior. Low identification with the mother is a highly significant predictor of later aggression in boys. On the other hand, for girls, low identification with the father was a significant predictor of later aggression. Examination of the aggression scores of high, medium, and low identification subjects revealed that low identification with both parents is the most potent predictor of aggression, irrespective of the subject's sex. Thus the hypothesis that identification with parents in certain motor behaviors such as walking, eating, and talking, and in perceptions of body image would be related to aggressive behavior was substantiated. As seen in Table 4, these measures obtained from both parents independently and from children in the third-grade classroom were correlated significantly to aggression synchronously in the third grade and longitudinally to aggression in the 13th grade. These findings lend support to the idea that what is termed conscience or internalization of parental proscriptions not only is copying of moral precepts and guilt for transgressions but also is copying of manifest motor behavior of the socializing agent. As seen later this finding parallels the effect of modeling on TV.

The measure of sex-typed behavior, comprised of empirically determined sex preference for games and activities, was included to test the hypothesis that identification with a particular sex role is related to aggression. The data supported this hypothesis. A boy's preference for girl's games and activities was an indicator of lower aggression both synchronously and in later years. Boys' preference for girls' games and activities was inversely correlated with peer nominations of aggression both in the third and 13th grades. Although not statistically significant, preference by boys for boys' games and activities was also in the hypothesized direction: the greater the preference, the more the aggression both in the third and in the 13th grades. For girls no statistically significant relations occurred. The literature on aggression is monotonous in the consistency with which it reports sex differences in aggression both in animal and in human subjects. Males are more aggressive than are females, and the reasons for this sex difference have been attributed to the learning of sex-role stereotypes, to biological-hormonal variables, or to both (Bronson & Desjardin, 1968; Feshbach, 1970; Maccoby & Jacklin, 1971; Mark & Ervin, 1970; Mischel, 1970; Young, Goy, & Pheonix, 1964). The data in the current study concerning sex-role learning and aggression are not at all in harmony with the position of biological determinism as an explanation of more aggression in the human male. Rather, the present findings lend support to the position of cultural anthropologists (Alland, 1972; Montagu, 1968) that, although the capacity to acquire culture may be biologically determined, the manifestation of a particular behavior is contingent upon it being learned in that culture.

The present data indicate that at least a portion of the variance accounting for sex differences in aggression is probably culturally determined. Masculine and feminine preferences made as early as eight years of age influence aggressive behavior at that time and also 10 years later. What emerges from these findings is that when boys opt for feminine games and activities, the choice in itself seems to act as a suppressor of early and later aggression. Preference for feminine activities may simply be incompatible with aggressive responses. Further evidence bearing on these relationships is presented later when it is shown that when adult females prefer stereotyped masculine activities such behavior is positively related to aggression.

The possibility of the child's imitating aggressive behavior is not limited exclusively to behavior exhibited by parents. As Bandura (1969) points out, children will copy the behavior of any *significant model*. Thus it should not be surprising that the hypothesis that a preference for a diet of violent TV would influence aggressive behavior was substantiated by our data. For boys there are statistically significant synchronous and longitudinal correlations between preference for viewing violent TV in the third grade and aggressive behavior at that time and 10 years later. As the multiple regression analyses revealed, preference for TV violence is a good predictor of later aggression. The order in which the variables were entered reveals that a preference for watching TV violence was the second most "useful" third-grade variable in the prediction. It explained more of the variance than any other predictor except one, mobility orientation, which explains only slightly more. More important, for a causal analysis however, are the standardized regression coefficients in the final regression equation. Such a coefficient can be interpreted as the contribution of the predictor variable to "causing" the criterion variable independent of the other predictor variables. The coefficients in Table 2 show that a preference by boys for violent TV in the third grade is one of the two major contributors to 13th-grade aggression among the third-grade variables. This finding supports the hypothesis that a preference for watching violent TV in the third-grade time period is a cause of aggressive habits later in life independent of the other causal contributors studied in boys.*

Path Analysis. A more specialized technique for using multiple regression coefficients to estimate causal effects is path analysis (Heise, 1970). The path coefficients for television and aggression are shown in Figure 1. These coefficients are standardized regression coefficients. In other words, the path coefficient from third-grade TV to 13th-grade aggression is the coefficient of third-grade TV violence in a regression equation predicting 13th-grade aggression with third-grade aggression controlled. The obtained pattern of path coefficients adds further credence to the argument that watching violent TV contributes to the development of aggressive habits in boys.

One final analysis is introduced to cap the contention that continued viewing of violence on TV influences the aggressive behavior of young boys. Table 6 presents the mean peer-rated aggression score of boys in the 13th grade as a function of their aggression score in the third grade and the preference for TV

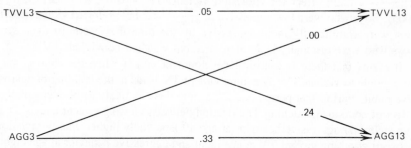

Figure 1. A path analysis indicating the dependencies between aggression and the viewing of violent TV for boys. The coefficients indicate the relative causal contributions of one variable to another. From L. D. Eron, L. R. Huesmann, M. M. Lefkowitz, & L. O. Walder. Does television violence cause aggression? *American Psychologist*, 1972, **27**(4), 260. Copyright 1972 by the American Psychological Association. Reprinted by permission.

*Two cross validations of these findings were done. The original multivariate analysis had been based on data from 128 boys and 120 girls. These included all subjects for whom there were complete data, that is, a score on every independent and dependent variable. In the first cross validation, all 427 subjects were included whether or not they had a score on every variable. The second cross validation used a 50% random sample of those subjects in the first cross validation. Those variables that appeared on the original regression analysis and held up on both cross validations are termed as of excellent validity; those that held up on one cross validation are termed fair; those that appeared on neither cross validation are termed as of poor validity. For boys, TV violence and nurturance are of excellent validity; identification with mother, preference for girls' games, and mobility orientation of parents are of fair validity; ethnicity is of poor validity. For girls, parents' religiosity and child's guilt are of excellent validity; TV violence, identification with father, and father's occupation, education and mobility orientation are of fair validity; IQ is of poor validity.

Table 6. Mean Aggression Score of Boys in 13th Grade as a Function of Aggression Score and Television in Third Grade

Level of Peer Rated Aggression in Third Grade	Preference for Television Violence in 3rd Grade			
	High	Medium	Low	
High	165.8 (13)[a]	116.9 (22)	60.6 (5)	114.4 (45)
Medium	103.3 (15)	89.3 (59)	58.7 (17)	83.9 (91)
Low	110.8 (8)	19.0 (31)	32.4 (9)	54.1 (43)
	126.6 (36)	75.1.(117)	50.6 (31)	

Source: L. R. Huesmann, L. D. Eron, M. M. Lefkowitz, & L. W. Walder. Television violence and aggression: the causal effect remains. American Psychologist, 1973, 28(7), 617-620. Copyright 1973 by the American Psychological Association. Reprinted by permission.
[a]Number in parentheses equals cell frequency.

violence in the third grade. As TV violence score increases, the 13th-grade aggression score also increases regardless of level of aggression in the third grade. There is a main effect for television violence $(F = 6.63, df = 2/175, p < .005)$. Boys who were low aggressive in grade three but preferred violent television were significantly more aggressive by the time they were 19 than were boys who were originally high aggressive but watched nonviolent TV.

It seems that there is a critical development period when the child is very susceptible to violent TV. Watching violent TV leads to the building of aggressive habits during that period and for a time there is likely to be a cumulative effect of continued watching. The relation between viewing violent television at age eight and aggressive behavior at age 19 is actually higher than the relation between watching violent TV at age eight and aggressive behavior at age eight. However, by the time the individual is 19 there is no longer a relation between the violence of what he views on television and how aggressive he is. Behavior patterns are already strongly established and the individual is no longer responsive to conditions which influence such behavior in the young.

When the boy is young—say between six and 12—and is continually bombarded with violence on television, he may well come to think this is a typical and therefore appropriate way to solve life's problems. We had the subjects at age 19 rate various Western and crime programs on how realistic they thought they were, for example, "How realistic do you think Gunsmoke is in telling about how life in the West really was?" or "How realistic would you say Mod Squad is in showing what police work is really like?" This scale we found was related to violence of programs preferred, the number of hours per week that television is watched and peer-rated aggression. That is, the more realistic these 19-year-old male subjects thought TV was, the more aggressive they were $(r = .34)$, the more they watched TV $(r = .28)$, and the more violent were the programs they preferred $(r = .36)$.

The Effects of TV Violence Upon Girls The differential availability on TV of aggressive male and female models, and the differential socialization practices to which girls are exposed, might limit the effect of TV violence on girls. The correlations in Table 4 support this view. There is a marginally significant negative relation between girls' preference for violent TV and aggressiveness in the 13th grade.

However, as pointed out previously, a multiple regression analysis can expose the causal contribution of each of several predictor variables to a dependent variable. If the effect of some predictor is being masked by other predictors, the regression analysis may expose it. Therefore, let us look at the regression equation for predicting girls' 13th-grade aggressiveness from the third-grade variables. The results of this analysis, displayed in Table 3, indicate that viewing TV violence may lead to *lessened* aggressiveness for girls. While the effect is not strong, it is significantly different from zero.

Why would TV violence affect girls this way? First, one must recognize that there are other hypotheses that could explain the regression besides the one which says that viewing violent TV reduces aggression in girls. Because there are no statistically significant bivariate correlations between girls' aggressiveness and their TV viewing habits, a cross-lagged analysis cannot be applied here to distinguish between rival hypotheses. However, a path analysis would be appropriate. The path analysis displayed in Figure 2 suggests both that early aggression leads to girls viewing less violent TV and that the continued viewing of violent TV leads to lessened aggression. This is a much weaker effect than that found for boys, and the lack of statistically significant bivariate relations makes us somewhat skeptical about pushing this theorizing too far. Nevertheless, let us try to explain why the viewing of violent TV, which clearly leads to heightened aggression in boys, might lead to lessened aggression in girls.

First, boys are often encouraged and reinforced in the direct and overt expression of aggression. On the other hand, girls are trained not to express aggres-

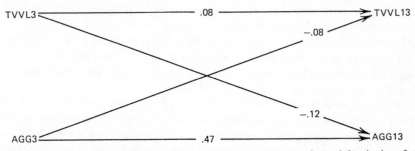

Figure 2. A path analysis indicating the dependencies between aggression and the viewing of violent TV for girls. The coefficients indicate the relative causal contributions of one variable to another.

sion in a direct manner and nonaggressive behaviors are reinforced. Thus for girls, TV violence viewing may actually be a positively sanctioned social activity in which aggressive girls may express their aggression vicariously. Second, there are far fewer aggressive females on TV for a girl to imitate than there are aggressive males for a boy to imitate. Also girls are victims on TV, not perpetrators. So the more violent the programs girls watch, the more they are exposed to female models as victims and the more they feel the aversive consequences of aggression. Therefore, violent TV would lead to less aggression in girls.

The suggestion that girls are trained not to express aggression in a direct manner relates to findings having to do with viewing of TV contact sports. The hypothesis that preference for viewing contact sports on TV would be related to aggressive behavior was substantiated, but only for girls $(r = .33, p < .01)$. Again, the rationale is offered that watching contact sports is a socially sanctioned activity in which the more aggressive girls may express agressive behavior vicariously.

Less restraint is placed on boys' expression of aggression so that the need for such vicarious channels would seem considerably less than that of girls. Indeed boys are frequently socially reinforced by adults and peers for the straightforward expression of aggression (Eron et al., 1971; Feshbach, 1970). Direct avenues for the expression of aggressive behavior such as fighting, wrestling, pummeling, and war games are open to boys but discouraged for girls. Moreover, both peer and adult cultures encourage and reinforce direct rather than vicarious participation for boys in contact sports but make little provision for the direct participation of girls. Thus for boys, knowledgeability of these sports is virtually peer-mandated and required for peer-acceptance and popularity.

A concomitant finding was that of a significant correlation for girls $(r = .18, p < .01)$ between peer nominations for aggression and scores in the direction of a masculine interest pattern as measured by Scale 5 of the MMPI. Thus results of the present study indicate that when females are aggressive, some of their interests and activities are deviant from that of their sex group, and they are similar in behavior to the male sex group. As counterpoint, the inverse relationships found for boys between aggression and preference for girls' games and activities in the third grade deserve repeating. The data indicate that low-aggressive males take on certain characteristics of females and high-aggressive females take on certain characteristics of males.

We have already suggested that the lack of aggressive female models on TV in 1960 would mitigate against girls identifying with an aggressive model. In addition we suggest that the girls who were eight years old in 1960 had been trained not to aggress openly, since aggression is considered to be unladylike. We also have evidence of this training, which is discussed later, where some sociocultural variables had quite different effects on boys and girls (e.g., church attendance). We propose that girls have been conditioned by society to express their aggression in a few socially acceptable forms and that fantasy is one of them. In fact, fantasy may be the only acceptable avenue for girls' aggressive behaviors. It is well known that young girls have greater verbal fluency, read better, and are better able to fantasize than boys. Thus girls may use violent TV fantasies to express their aggressions and then aggress less in situations in which their peers see them.

What support can we marshall for this theory? Recent research by Singer (1972) has revealed that children can relieve aggression by viewing aggressive acts if they have been trained to distinguish reality from fantasy. Thus if our theorizing is correct, one would expect girls to be able to distinguish reality from fantasy in TV programs better than boys could. Data we collected in the 13th grade confirm just this. Girls think television is significantly less realistic than do boys $(t = 1.706, df = 425, p < .05)$. Given this finding, one can check some other implications of this theory. Assuming that girls who think TV is realistic would be poor fantasizers, one would expect to find them in the higher aggression groups. One can see from Table 7 that this is exactly the case. Finally, we note that girls who see themselves as masculine in the 13th grade, that is, who obtain high scores on Scale 5 of the MMPI, tend to perceive TV as more realistic and tend to be more aggressive in situations where their peers can see them. The correlations between MMPI Scale 5 and "realism on TV" was .22, while the correlation betwen MMPI Scale 5 and peer-rated aggression was .18. In summary, while it is not completely clear from our data that viewing TV violence reduces peer-rated aggression scores for girls, the reasons why girls might express their aggressions by watching violent TV programs seem plausible.

Amount of TV Viewing. While the amount of TV viewing a boy engages in at eight is not related to his later aggressiveness, it is negatively correlated with his concurrent aggressiveness $(r = -.19)$. The more aggressive a boy is at age eight, the less TV he watches. One might hypothesize that boys who act nonaggressively stay home and watch TV, perhaps to avoid aggressive encounters. However, an alternative explanation that we find more tenable is that boys who stay home and watch TV are aggressive at home and are not seen as being aggressive as frequently by their peers. We find this later hypothesis more appealing, since the aggression of the child as rated by the mother was positively correlated with the amount of TV watching $(r = .24)$ and also since aggression anxiety, which should be high if a boy is extremely *nonaggressive,* was not high for the boys who watched a lot of TV. The amount of TV a girl watches is mostly unrelated to her aggressiveness.

Sociocultural Variables

While generally the sociocultural variables were good predictors of a child's aggression in the third and 13th grades, several were inconsistent. However, one

Table 7. Mean Score for Girls on Judged "Realism of TV Programs" As a Function of Girls' Aggressiveness in Third and 13th Grades

Aggression Classification	Realism Score	
	Third Grade	13th Grade
Low	12.65	13.77
Medium	15.58	15.91
High	17.50	19.10
	$F = 2.33$	$F = 4.07$
	$df = 2/213$	$df = 2/213$
	$p < .041$	$p < .018$

consistent predictor of aggression was socioeconomic status as measured by the father's occupation. High status occupations were designated by a low number so the multiple regressions indicate that a child's aggressiveness increases as father's occupational status increases. This effect is highly significant for daughters at both the third and 13th grades, but only at the third grade for sons. Furthermore, in this same general context of socioeconomic status, parents' upward social mobility orientation was a good predictor to aggressive behavior at age 19 for both boys and girls. Social mobility as measured in the present study was contingent upon movement, change, and continuing demands for adjustments to new situations. These kinds of behaviors are similar to instigators of aggression in that they characterize a fluid and unstable situation that is conceivably frustrating to children.

The conventional view that aggression is a positive trait associated with ambition, with the entrepreneurial spirit, and with such events as discovery and the technological advancement of a society are actually supported by these findings. If the child's aspirations and achievements were correlated with those of his parents, then aggressive behavior might be positively associated with high occupational aspirations, achievement of high occupational status, and upward social mobility. Data from the longitudinal phase of the present study tend to support such an hypothesis. A total self-aspiration score comprised of educational, financial, and occupational aspiration was computed for each of the 13th-grade subjects. For both sexes the correlations between 13th-grade peer-rated aggression, and this total aspiration score were positive and in the hypothesized direction (males: $r = .36, p < .01$; females: $r = .14, p < .10$). Thus not only is parents' striving for material accomplishments related to their children's aggression, but also, as these children mature, their own desire for material success is positively associated with aggressiveness.

While higher occupational status of her father was found to be predictive of higher aggression in a girl, higher parental educational status was associated with lower aggression in girls both in the third grade and 10 years later. This finding appears to repeat our earlier discovery in which significant negative correlations were obtained between achievement test scores in high-school and 13th-grade aggression. Low school achievement was interpreted to be an instigator of aggression. In the same manner, low education of parents may be viewed as an instigator of aggression in their daughters. It may simply be the case that poorly educated parents are unaware of those child-rearing techniques which serve to mitigate aggressiveness, and so they create an environment which contains more frustrating situations for their daughters than do well-educated parents.

Parents' frequency of church attendance appears to have a differential effect upon their sons' and daughters' aggressiveness. The more the parents reported they attended church when the subjects were eight years old, the less was the aggressiveness of their daughters 10 years later. For boys, however, there was no relation. These results may be indicative of differential socialization practices. Parents may attempt to inculcate church teachings to "love your enemies" and "turn the other cheek" in training their daughters to respond to aggression. Since nonaggression is "ladylike" and expected of girls, such training is consonant with church doctrine. For boys, just the opposite in socialization practices is often the case. For boys to respond to aggression with counteraggression is seen as manly, and to "turn the other cheek" is viewed as craven. Recall that these subjects were raised in the period of the early 1950s when the notion of unisex and women's liberation were not widely known. Expectations of boys were that they behave like men, and, if anything, training in the direct expression of aggression was the rule. Thus if nonaggression as a principle was promulgated by the church, it may have had less relevance to the socialization of boys than of girls.

It is noteworthy that in Western Christian countries a close association exists between soldiering and masculinity. Women may enlist or be drafted for noncombatant positions—in the main clerical and nursing—but Christian societies would view with opprobrium the suggestion that women directly "man" the weapons of death and destruction. Whereas, the opposite is true for men. Opposition to the Equal Rights Amendment in the United States has largely been on this basis.

However, there are indications that socialization of young girls may be changing. Current research with nine-year-old boys and girls (Chiswick, 1973) indicates that girls now, for the first time in our studies over the past 15 years, are obtaining scores just as high as boys in an experimental situation in which overt aggressive behavior is measured. Concurrently, we note that in the last five or six years, while these nine-year-old girls have been increasingly exposed to TV, there have been increasingly more aggressive females whose behavior could be copied, for example, "Mod Squad," "Ironside," and "Girl from

UNCLE.'' This is not to say one is causing the other. Both may be a function of the rapidly changing role of women in our society.

To summarize results with aggression, the data collected on the four classes of independent variables have shown a variety of important relationships to the development of aggression. The patterning of the relations indicates that certain socialization practices called instigators, such as rejection, have their greatest effect on aggressive behavior during the period of childhood but that the effect does not extend into young adulthood. Other variables, however, such as modeling and sociocultural factors influence aggressive behavior synchronously and also across time. Sex of subject was another dimension in which patterning differences occurred. For example, preference for violent TV programs significantly influenced boys' aggressive behavior in the third and 13th grades, whereas girls' behavior was influenced in the opposite direction in the 13th grade. Similarly preference for viewing televised contact sports was positively associated with 13th-grade aggression, but only for females, and, as noted, parents' church attendance was related to girls' aggression but not to boys' aggression.

The aggression measures themselves were substantially correlated across time, indicating that aggression as measured in childhood is a good predictor of aggression in young adulthood and that this is a fairly stable characteristic. In addition, the peer-nomination measure of aggresssion was significantly correlated with other measures of aggression obtained in the 13th grade.

RESULTS AND DISCUSSION—PSYCHOPATHOLOGY

It was stated at the beginning of this chapter that aggression was assumed to be one aspect of emotional health and that the learning conditions which were propaedeutic to the appearance of hostile behavior would be similar to the antecedents of other types of maladaptive behavior. Unfortunately no direct measures of emotional disturbance or psychopathology were included for the subjects when they were eight years old; thus causal analysis of the data was difficult. One index to emotional disturbance that was used was admission of subjects to state hospitals in New York. However, only three of the 427 subjects had a record of having been admitted to a state hospital in New York before 1971. This is not surprising, since there are relatively few young persons admitted to such institutions (New York State Department of Mental Hygiene, 1972). Also this is a relatively insensitive index to presence of psychopathology, since only severely disturbed individuals get admitted to such institutions and in addition there are social class and regional biases affecting admission rates. However, in the 13th grade each subject was administered a personality inventory, the MMPI (Hathaway and McKinley, 1969), probably a more sensitive instrument to detect psychopathology than state hospital admissions. As an indication of psychopathology we used the sum of scores on the psychotic tetrad (scales 6,

7, 8, and 9, labeled paranoia, psychasthenia, schizophrenia, and hypomania, respectively). There is evidence that this is a valid index to potential and actual psychotic behavior (Dahlstrom, Welsh & Dahlstrom, 1972).

Boys

Although aggression and psychopathology scores are related (as discussed later in this chapter), the antecedent variables we have been discussing have quite a different relation to psychopathology than to aggression. Whereas instigators, contingent response, identification, and social class were related to aggression contemporaneously, only the latter two related to aggression over a 10-year time span. For prediction of psychopathology at age 19, however, the opposite is true. This is seen in Table 8 which lists all those variables, measured when the subjects were eight years old, which are significantly related to the MMPI psychotic tetrad scores at age 19. For boys, rejection by father at age eight is the parent variable most closely related to the psychopathology score at age 19. Rejection by mother is also related to the psychopathology score. However, as Table 9 reveals, the average psychopathology score for boys varies significantly only with father's rejection, not mother's ($F = 5.116$, $df = 2/131$, $p < .008$). This pattern of means reveals something that is masked by the correlation

Table 8. Correlations between Third-Grade Antecedent Variables and the MMPI Psychotic Tetrad Scores [a]

Variable	Females	Males
Aggression, third grade	.091	.138
Aggression anxiety	−.076	−.269
Preference for girls' games	−.177	.081
Father's occupation	.153	.052
Father's rejection	.153	.242
Mother's rejection	.014	.172
Father's rating of home aggression	−.059	.180
Mother's rating of home aggression	−.030	.153
Confessing	−.078	−.172
Mother's punishment	.153	−.056
Father's acquiescence	.208	−.015
Mother's education	.190	.054
TV hours watched	.162	.066
IQ	−.099	−.233
Punishment, mother and father	.138	−.134
Rejection, mother and father	.119	.229
Aggression, 13th grade [b]	.120	.276

[a]This table includes every antecedent (third grade) variable for which there is a significant univariate correlation with the Tetrad score for either males or females.

[b]This is not a third-grade antecedent variable but is included for illustrative purposes.

Table 9.   Mean Scores on Psychotic Tetrad of MMPI 1 As a Function of Various Levels of Rejection

	Boys				Girls			
	Mother				Mother			
Father	LO	MED	HI	TOTAL	LO	MED	HI	TOTAL
LO	245.10	233.86	245.29	241.42	228.69	235.58	219.20	227.82
MED	230.80	230.60	239.69	233.70	228.24	236.45	213.71	226.13
HI	276.16	252.43	256.01	261.53	223.21	239.44	240.36	234.34
TOTAL	250.68	238.96	247.09	245.55	226.72	237.16	224.42	229.43

coefficient. The greatest difference in psychopathology scores is between those subjects whose parents score moderately high on the rejection scale and those who score very high. The difference between the high- and low-rejection groups was not significant. An examination of the content of the rejection scale suggests a reasonable interpretation for this finding. The rejection items deal with behaviors in the child which the parent feels are worthy of change, for example, "Do you think Johnny is too forgetful?" "Are you satisfied with Johnny's manners?" "Are you pleased with the quality of Johnny's schoolwork?" Parents who have very low scores on this scale, indicating that they feel their child is perfect, are probably communicating unrealistic evaluations to their child. Parents in the medium classification, indicating there are some areas in which the child can improve his behavior, are communicating a more realistic image; while parents with high scores are saying the child can never measure up to their standards, thus communicating a very negative evaluation. The same pattern holds for both mothers and fathers. Thus it would seem that parents in the moderate range on this rejection scale are setting up reasonable expectations for their children, training them not to expect universal approval from everyone they interact with, but also not encouraging a defeatist attitude about their competencies. It would seem that a little rejection has positive effects. This has also been demonstrated in a study relating child-rearing practices to creativity in children (Siegelman, 1973).

Of the child variables, aggression anxiety and IQ are most closely related to psychopathology, both negatively, so that the lower the male child's IQ and the less anxious he is about aggression at age eight, the more disturbed is his behavior 10 years later. There is a much smaller positive relation between how aggressive the boy is at age eight, as rated by his peers, and his psychopathology score at age 19. The relation is much more marked between his peer-rated aggression score at age 19 and his psychopathology score at that time.

Identification variables also predict psychopathology. The more the parent says his son confesses at age eight, the less psychopathological are his scores on the MMPI 10 years later. Confessing, it will be recalled, was one measure of internalization of standards. However, confessing behavior might also be an indication of warmth and acceptance by the parent. The child who feels he can confess misdeeds freely to his parents is likely to have a warm relationship with them.

Modest positive relations to psychopathology were also obtained with ratings of aggressive behavior at home when the child was eight years old. The ratings were made by both mother and father. It is interesting that these positive correlations between home aggression at age eight and psychopathology at age 19 are as large as those between home aggression at age eight and peer-rated aggression at age 19. (The latter correlation was .20 for mothers and .12 for fathers.) Also the correlations between home aggression and psychopathology are larger than the correlation between home aggression and peer-rated aggression when both are measured at age eight. (The latter correlation was .001 for mothers and .13 for fathers.) Perhaps the rating of aggression at home, made by the parents when these boys were eight years old, served also as an indirect measure of how disturbed the parent felt the child was. Parents for whom aggressive behavior on the part of the child was salient possibly saw this as a manifestation of maladaptive behavior. In support of this hypothesis there is a moderate relation between peer-rated aggression at age 19 and self-rating for psychopathology among male subjects $(r = .28)$. The pattern of these relations gives us more confidence in the proposition that aggression is an aspect of psychopathology, as stated in the beginning of this chapter. Furthermore, the variables which we termed instigators to aggression in the third grade, while not related to aggression 10 years later, are related to the appearance of psychopathology in the later period.

The multiple regression analysis, which, as pointed out previously in discussing the prediction of aggression, can give an estimate of the relative causal contribution of antecedent variables to a criterion, indicates (Table 10) that an important antecedent factor to psychopathology in males at age 19 is indeed rejection by parents (a score which is summed for mothers and fathers). However, the most important factor to emerge in this regression analysis is contingent response to aggression which is related negatively, so that low punishment goes with increased disturbance. Both of these variables reflect a minimal amount of interaction with the child. The parent who doesn't punish his son for transgressions is perhaps communicating that he doesn't really care about him, and, in the same way as the rejecting parent does, also tends to discourage interaction between parent and child. It is in these early interchanges with his parents that the child practices interpersonal skills and learns how to evaluate his own behavior and its effects on others. Persons who score high on the psychopathology scales do not do these things well. Thus it is not surprising that IQ also has a causal contribution, since duller children have fewer resources for interpersonal skills. Furthermore, it is interesting that the peer-rating measure of aggression anxiety taken at age eight has by itself the highest correlation to the MMPI

Table 10.   Multiple Regression Analyses Predicting MMPI Psychotic Tetrad

Third-Grade Predictor	Females			Males		
Variable	Standard-ized Coefficient	Signifi-cance	Unique Variance	Standard-ized Coefficient	Signifi-cance	Unique Variance
Preference for girls' games	−.179	.05	.032			
Aggression anxiety				−.272	.002	.066
Punishment				−.302	.001	.078
IQ				−.200	.019	.037
Rejection				.193	.025	.034
	$F = 3.09$	$df = 3/185$	$p < .01$	$F = 6.37$	$df = 5/122$	$p < .001$

measure of psychopathology in male subjects and is the second most important predictor in the multiple regression analysis. Boys who are anxious about expressing aggression at age eight tend *not* to have high MMPI psychopathology scores at age 19. The items in the aggression anxiety scale reflect a tendency to try to facilitate interpersonal relations ("Who says excuse me even when they have not done anything bad?" "Who will never fight even when picked on?"). Such boys care about their interactions with others and have probably learned techniques which help them get along well with others. Consequently they are more apt to gain gratifications from interpersonal relations and will not develop the maladaptive, defensive behaviors which are tapped by the MMPI items.*

Girls

For girls the patterns of correlations (Table 8) and the regression analysis (Table 10) reveal a somewhat different pattern of causal contribution of parent variables and other measures taken in the third grade to psychopathology at age 19. The most striking difference is that there is no relation between peer-rated aggression anxiety and the psychotic tetrad for girls, nor between peer-rated aggression and that psychopathology score. One possible reason for the difference is that the types of behavior reflected by the aggression anxiety score are learned by most girls very early in life and approximate the norm of behavior for girls. Thus these behaviors are probably not related to individual differences in the ability to get along with others, as they are in boys.

Another difference is the direct relation between social class status of family

*The cross validations performed subsequent to the derivation of the multiple regression equation, as described in footnote on p. 71, indicated that fair validity would be ascribed to rejection and punishment while aggression anxiety and IQ were of excellent validity.

at age eight years and psychopathology at age 19 which obtains for girls but not for boys. The lower the social class as measured both by father's occupation and mother's education when the girl was eight, the greater is the tendency towards high scores on the psychotic tetrad. However, for boys there was no relation between psychopathology score and any of the social status indices. Father's acquiescence (a measure taken from the F scale), which has the highest relation to the psychotic tetrad for girls, is highly related to social class (Christie, Havel, & Seidenberg. 1958).

Two variables having more to do with recreational than occupational activities are important antecedents to psychopathology for girls. Girls who prefer boys' games at age eight and girls who spend more time watching TV during that period are the ones who develop more maladaptive ways of behaving than do girls who prefer the appropriate sex-typed recreational activities. Engaging in role inappropriate behavior at age eight is an indicator of later psychopathology and perhaps is the reason for the positive correlation between punishment for aggression at age eight and score on the psychotic tetrad. The size of the bivariate correlation is the same as for boys, although it is in the opposite direction. Aggression is an inappropriate behavior for girls. Parents who say they punish their daughters severely for this behavior are perhaps responding to that expectation and are already taking note of this deviance and labeling it for us. It is interesting that it is only this parental response to aggression which is related to psychopathology in female subjects. Neither aggression at home as rated by either parent, or aggression in school as rated by peers, in the third grade and again in the 13th grade are correlated with psychopathology. In the multiple regression analysis, girls' third-grade peer-rated aggression is the second variable to enter the analysis explaining slightly more than 2% of the variance, and the father's aggression as measured by the Walters and Zak scale (1959) enters as the third variable explaining slightly less than 2%. Neither one of these coefficients however is significant at the .05 level of confidence.*

Thus at least from this analysis it would seem that the original assumption that aggression is one aspect of psychopathology does not hold up as well for females as it does for male children. Furthermore, some of the same learning conditions which are antecedent to aggression in males lead to psychopathology in girls. A more direct way of observing this is to note the number of significant correlations between the 10 MMPI scales and the 43 variables derived from the parent interview. For girls there are 90 significant correlations and for boys, 62, out of a total number of 559 correlations for each of the two groups. This difference is highly significant (chi square = 5.157).

*In the cross validations described previously nonpreference for girls' games and activities was of excellent validity as a predictor to psychotic tetrad scores. Peer-rated aggression at grade 3 was of fair validity and father's aggression was of poor validity.

Discriminant Function Analysis

Another way of looking at the relation between psychopathology and aggression is to separate the sample of subjects into high-aggressive and low-aggressive groups and do a discriminant function analysis between the two groups, predicting by use of correlation coefficients from each of the 13 MMPI scales (three validity and 10 clinical scales) to the aggression categorization. This was done separately for boys and girls and for aggression at ages eight and 19. Subjects in the upper and lower quartiles of peer-rated aggression at each of these periods were used in the analysis. Additional analyses were done for those subjects who were classified in the same quartiles (upper or lower) at both periods. Because intelligence and social class have in the past been related to scores on the MMPI (Dahlstrom et al., 1972) these two variables were also entered into the discriminant function analysis.

In the analysis of the data for male subjects using aggression scores at age eight, the overall test for no difference in means yielded a significant F $(F = 3.172, df = 15/92; p < .01)$. Thus it is possible to examine the individual t tests for their contributions to the discrimination between the high- and low-aggressive subjects. Four of the 15 scales discriminate between the two groups: intelligence (low-aggressive boys have higher IQ scores); hypochondriasis (low-aggressive boys have a higher number of physical complaints); psychopathic deviate (high-aggressive boys have a greater tendency toward antisocial behavior); and psychasthenia (low-aggressive boys have more obsessive-compulsive defenses).

Using peer-rated aggression at age 19 to separate the boys into high- and low-aggression groups, the overall test again yielded a significant F $(F = 4.362, df = 15/95; p < .001)$. Individual scales contributing to the discrimination between low- and high-aggressive boys at age 19 were the k scale (low-aggressive males endorsing more socially acceptable behaviors); the psychopathic deviate scale (high-aggressive males again tending more towards antisocial behavior); and psychasthenia (low-aggressive males again utilizing more obsessive compulsive defenses).

When we compare males who are high on peer-rated aggression both at ages eight and 19 with males low in aggression at both times, the discriminant function analysis again yielded an overall significant F $(F = 3.549, df = 15/32; p < .01)$. The discriminating scales were intelligence (low-aggressive boys had higher IQ scores); hypochondriasis (low-aggressive males have more hypochondriacal complaints); psychasthenia (low-aggressive males have more obsessive compulsive defenses); and schizophrenia (high-aggressive males admit to more schizophrenic-like behaviors). It is quite apparent from these results that aggression can indeed be called a facet of psychopathology.

For females the discriminant function analysis relating third-grade aggression and MMPI scale scores at age 8 yielded a significant overall F $(F = 3.064,$

$df = 15/103; p < .01$). The discriminating scales were intelligence (low-aggressive females have higher IQ scores); masculinity (high-aggressive females are more masculine in interests, attitudes, and behaviors); and social isolation (low-aggressive girls tend to withdraw from social interaction more than high-aggressive girls).

The discriminant function analysis for females relating peer-rated aggression scores at age 19 to MMPI scales again yielded a significant F ($F = 3.788$, $df = 15/96; p < .01$). Two scales contributed to this discrimination: F (with high-aggressive females saying more unusual things about themselves); and psychopathic deviate (with high-aggressive females tending more toward antisocial behavior).

When we compare females who ae high on peer-rated aggression both at ages eight and 19 with females low in aggression at both times, the discriminant function analysis yielded an overall significant F ($F = 3.108$, $df = 15/41; p < .01$). However, only one scale contributed to this discrimination: social isolation (with low-aggressive girls tending more to withdrawal from interpersonal relations).

To summarize results obtained from the discriminant function analysis, it is apparent that there is a strong relation between the aggression level of both female and male subjects (so classified by a peer-nomination measure), and the manner in which these subjects endorse items on a set of scales measuring psychopathological deviance. However, there are more such relations between psychopathology and aggression for males than for females. High-aggressive males are more prone to engage in antisocial and other deviant behaviors; low-aggressive males are more likely to develop hypochondriacal complaints and obsessive compulsive symptoms. High-aggressive females are more masculine in their attitudes and interests, and low-aggressive females tend more to withdraw from social interaction than high-aggressive females. In both males and females higher aggression is associated with lower intelligence. It should be emphasized, however, that the effect of IQ is independent of the other scales in this analysis which accounts for the unique contribution of each variable to the criterion.

SUMMARY

In this chapter we have described a 10-year follow-up study relating learning conditions provided by parents at home to the aggressive behavior of their children. Learning conditions were assessed when the children were in the third grade, and their aggressive behavior was measured at that time and then again 10 years later. Aggression had been assumed to be an aspect of mental health; thus at the 10-year follow-up, a measure of psychopathology (the psychotic tetrad score on the MMPI) was also obtained from the subjects.

The learning conditions from which predictions were made to behavior 10 years later included four types of variables: instigation; reinforcement; identification; and social class. While all four kinds of antecedents had related to aggression concurrently when the children were in the third grade, only identification and social class were related to aggressive behavior 10 years later. Of the identification variables, the most important was the models of behavior furnished on the childrens' favorite TV programs.

As for psychopathology, it was demonstrated that aggression does seem to be related to mental health as originally assumed. Furthermore, variables classified as instigators, especially rejection, which did not relate to aggressive behavior over the 10-year time span did relate to psychopathology. Punishment and identification were also related to psychopathology, as was social class.

There were consistent differences in findings for boys and girls in the relation of the antecedent variables both to aggression and psychopathology. In many cases the learning conditions which lead to aggression in boys were related to psychopathology in girls. The differences were ascribed to differential socialization of boys and girls.

REFERENCES

Alland, A., Jr. *The human imperative*. New York: Columbia University Press, 1972.

Azrin, N. H. Some effects of noise on human behavior. *Journal of Experimental Analysis of Behavior*, 1958, **1**, 183–200.

Bandura, A. *Principles of behavior modification*. New York: Holt, Rinehart, & Winston, 1969.

Bandura, A., Ross, D., & Ross, S. Imitation of film mediated aggressive models. *Journal of Abnormal Psychology*, 1963a, **66**, 3–11.

Bandura, A., Ross, D., & Ross, S. Vicarious reinforcement and imitative learning. *Journal of Abnormal Psychology*, 1963b, **67**, 601–607.

Bandura, A., & Walters, R. H. *Social learning and personality development*. New York: Holt, 1963.

Bronson, F. H., & Desjardins. Aggression in adult mice: Modification by neonatal injections of gonadal hormones. *Science*, 1968, **161**, 705–706.

Chasdi, E. H., & Lawrence, M. S. Some antecedents of aggression and effects of frustration in doll play. In D. McClelland (Ed.), *Studies in motivation*. New York: Appleton-Century-Crofts, 1955.

Chiswick, N. An experimental study of the effects of punishment and permission on aggression and anxiety. Unpublished doctoral dissertation, University of Illinois at Chicago Circle, 1973.

Christie, R., Havel, J., & Seidenberg, B. Is the F scale irreversible? *Journal of Abnormal and Social Psychology*, 1958, **56**, 143–159.

Dahlstrom, W. G., Welsh, G. S., & Dahlstrom, L. E. *An MMPI handbook*. Vol. 1. *Clinical interpretation*. Minneapolis: University of Minnesota Press, 1972.

Darlington, R. D. Multiple regression in psychological research and practice. *Psychological Bulletin*, 1968, **64**, 161–182.

Eron, L. D., Huesmann, L. R., Lefkowitz, M. M. & Walder, L. O. Does television violence cause aggression? *American Psychologist*, 1972, **27**, 253–263.

Eron, L. D., Walder, L. O., & Lefkowitz, M. M. *Learning of aggression in children*. Boston: Little, Brown & Company, 1971.

Eron, L. D. Walder, L. O., Toigo, R., & Lefkowitz, M. M. Social class, parental punishment for aggression and child aggression. *Child Development*, 1963, **34**, 849–867.

Feshbach, S. Aggression. In P. H. Mussen (Ed.) *Carmichael's manual of child psychology*. Vol. 2. (3rd ed.) New York: Wiley, 1970. Pp. 159–250.

Feshbach, S., & Singer, R. D. *Television and aggression*. San Franc sco: Jossey-Bass, 1971.

Frank, G. H. Role of the family in the development of psychopathology. *Psychological Bulletin*, 1965, **64**, 191–205.

Freud, S. *The ego and the id*. London: Hogarth Press, 1923.

Greenberg, B. S., & Gordon, T. F. Perceptions of violence in television programs: Critics and the public. In G. A. Comstock & E. A. Rubinstein (Eds.), *Television and social behavior*. Vol. 1. *Content and control*. Washington, D.C.: Government Printing Office, 1971.

Hathaway, S. R., & McKinley, J. C. *The Minnesota multiphasic personality inventory*. New York: The Psychological Corporation, 1969.

Hathaway, S. R., & Monachesi, E. D. *An atlas of juvenile MMPI profiles*. Minneapolis: University of Minnesota Press, 1961.

Heise, D. R. Causal inference from panel data. In E. F. Borgatta & G. W. Bohrnstedt (Eds.) *Sociological methodology 1970*. San Francisco: Jossey-Bass, 1970.

Lefkowitz, M. M. Some relationships between sex role preference of children and other parent-child variables. *Psychological Reports*, 1962, **10**, 43–53.

Lefkowitz, M. M., Eron, L. D., Walder, L. O., & Huesmann, L. R. Television violence and child aggression: A follow-up study. In G. A. Comstock and E. A. Rubenstein, *Television and social behavior*. Vol. 3. *Adolescent aggressiveness*. Washington, D.C.: U.S. Government Printing Office, 1971. Pp. 35–135.

Maccoby, E. E., & Jacklin, C. N. Sex differences and their implications for sex roles. Paper presented at meetings of American Psychological Association, Washington, D.C., 1971.

Mark, V., & Ervin, F. *Violence and the brain*. New York: Harper and Row, 1970.

Mischel, W. Sex typing and socialization. In P. H. Mussen (Ed.), *Carmichael's manual of child psychology*. Vol. 2. (3rd ed.) New York: Wiley, 1970.

Montagu, M. F. A. The new litany of "innate depravity" or original sin revisited. In M. F. A. Montagu, *Man and aggression*. New York: Oxford University Press, 1968. Pp. 3–17.

Orlansky, H. Infant care and personality. *Psychological Bulletin,* 1949, **46,** 1–48.

Osgood, C. E., Suci, G. J., & Tannenbaum, P. H. *The measurement of meaning.* Urbana, Illinois: University of Illinois Press, 1957.

Semler, I. J., & Eron, L. D. Replication report: Relationship of aggression in third grade children to certain pupil characteristics. *Psychology in the Schools,* 1967, **4,** 356–358.

Siegelman, M. Parent behavior correlates of personality traits related to creativity in sons and daughters. *Journal of Consulting and Clinical Psychology,* 1973, **40,** 43–47.

Singer, J. L. *The child's world of make believe: Experimental studies of imaginative play.* New York: Academic Press, 1972.

Sullivan, E. T., Clark, W. W., & Tiegs, E. W. *California short form test of mental maturity.* Los Angeles: California Test Bureau, 1957.

Toigo, R. Parental social status as a contextual and individual determinant of aggressive behavior among third grade children in the classroom situation. Unpublished doctoral dissertation, Columbia University, 1962.

Walder, L. O., Abelson, R., Eron, L. D., Banta, T. J., & Laulicht, J. H. Development of a peer-rating measure of aggression. *Psychological Reports,* 1961, **9,** 497–556 (monograph supplement 4-49).

Walters, R. H., & Zak, M. S. Validation studies of an aggression scale. *Journal of Psychology,* 1959, **47,** 209–218.

Warner, W. L., Meeker, M., & Eells, K. *Social class in America.* New York: Harcourt, 1960.

Young, W. C., Goy, R. W., & Pheonix, C. H. Hormones and sexual behavior. *Science,* 1964, **143,** 212–218.

CHAPTER 3

Phobias of Childhood in a Prescientific Era

LOVICK C. MILLER, CURTIS L. BARRETT, AND EDWARD HAMPE

Phobias have been observed at every age in man except shortly after birth, within all cultures, and through all recorded history. Hippocrates described two adults, one with a fear of the notes of a flute and the other with a fear of heights. Despite the fact that fears and phobias have plagued man since the earliest of time and have been studied extensively since the turn of this century, phobias remain a mystery. In fact, we are in a most peculiar situation, for we know that phobias exist, that they can be excessively painful and can severely interrupt and cripple a person's life, and yet we have no adequate theory to explain their presence nor predict their future, no reliable instruments to measure their presence or their progress, very little sophisticated research, and no generally agreed upon definition. Berecz concluded his review of the literature as follows: "There is presently too little empirical evidence in the area of childhood phobias to allow many meaningful generalizations [1968, pp. 714–715]."

Since we find the same state of affairs in 1974, we have entitled our chapter, "Phobias of Childhood in a Prescientific Era." In the chapter, we plan to acquaint the reader with the relevant questions in the study of childhood phobia, the experience of others, as well as our own, in dealing with these questions, and a consensus of the current state of the treatment art. In taking this approach, we are making no claim to have exhausted the literature, nor to have generated sophisticated critiques of theory. Rather, we have asked ourselves what are the constantly recurring issues in the study and treatment of phobia that clinicians and researchers confront, and what is the residue of their experience which, in lieu of scientific knowledge, can be considered the "conventional wisdom."

DEFINITION

When we attempt to define the phenomenon, the complexity of our subject is illustrated immediately. The primary issue involves the distinction between fear and phobia. Fear is commonly thought of as the normal physiological reaction to genuine threat, and it involves outer behavioral expressions, inner subjective feelings, and accompanying physiological changes. Phobia is a special type of fear in which responses are excessive, persistent, and unadaptive.

Thus fear is considered a reasonable response to frightening stimuli, while phobia is an unreasonable response, often to relatively benign or ill-defined stimuli. Aside from the problem of operationalizing the reasonableness of a response, more fundamental theoretical issues are involved. Social learning and behavior theorists have assumed that the unreasonable response is learned and make it their object of study, while psychoanalytic theorists maintain that the unreasonableness is a symptom of underlying unconscious processes, arising from instinctual conflicts. Developmental theorists argue that unreasonableness can only be understood within a developmental context; for example, separation anxiety in a nine-month-old is considered "reasonable," but is "unreasonable" in a 10-year-old. Transactional theorists contend that phobias are imbedded within an interpersonal relationship. Thus it follows that a definition is dependent upon theory, and without a generally acceptable theory, any definition must be arbitrary.

As a result of this conclusion we have arbitrarily selected and enlarged upon Marks' (1969) definition as follows: A phobia is a special form of fear which,

1. Is out of proportion to demands of the situation.
2. Cannot be explained or reasoned away.
3. Is beyond voluntary control.
4. Leads to avoidance of the feared situation.
5. Persists over an extended period of time.
6. Is unadaptive.
7. Is not age or stage specific.

This definition leaves out the concept of unconscious symbolization and the interactional component which are discussed in a later section.

CLASSIFICATION

The systematic classification of phobias began in the latter part of the nineteenth century. The first effort was to describe responses to stimuli and to label the *S-R* sequence with Greek names. Thus the Greek word "phobos" meant panic-fear and terror, and the prefix "agora" referred to open spaces; thus a fear of open spaces was termed "agoraphobia." This labeling process proliferated to the point of absurdity because almost any stimulus could elicit a phobic reaction (Berecz, 1968). It is now generally recognized that a classification scheme based upon the feared object will result in an endless terminology. However, no satisfactory alternative has as yet been proposed.

Since there is no generally accepted nosology of child phobia, we would like to propose one. In the construction of our nosology we have drawn primarily from research and clinical experience, rather than from theory. The criterion governing its construction was that it be clinically usable, that is, points to different treatments, yields prognoses, and shows the limit of current knowledge. The simplest scheme would be a school-phobic–other-phobic dichotomy. This appears absurd, yet our survey of the literature reveals that school phobia is unique in that it is the only phobic condition that has been studied extensively. The ratio of professional papers on school phobia to any other phobia is at least 25—1. Furthermore, school phobia is the main phobic condition referred for treatment. In our study of child phobia (Miller, Barrett, Hampe, & Noble, 1972a) we made every effort, over a 3-year period, to enlist all types of phobias. But we ended with 69% school-phobics, even though our surveys show that school phobia occurs in less than 1% of the general population, while other phobias run as high as 20%. School phobia is the phobia that most concerns parents and professionals. Thus it is not unreasonable to consider a simple dichotomous classification.

However, we believe that such a classification would obscure the main issues and impede further work. We also believe a more encompassing scheme is warranted. To create one, a reasonable grouping of phobic objects needs to be made. In addition, the age of the child, the chronicity of the phobia, the severity of the child's and family's disturbance, the conditioning history, and the reinforcements that maintain the phobia need to be taken into consideration.

Table 1 presents our proposed nosology. It is advanced tentatively, because very little reliable research has been done in this area. As research evidence accumulates, the scheme should be modified. This modification would be particularly true for the placement of specific phobic objects and the subclassifications within the major categories.

The first decision a clinician must make is whether the phobia is the primary problem or is secondary to a more pervasive condition. All major childhood syndromes such as aggression, hyperactivity, antisocial behavior, social withdrawal, learning disability, depression, or psychosis may feature phobias which are secondary to the major complaint. In such cases, the condition is classified as a *phobic state* within a more general disorder. Our scheme excludes these conditions. When the phobia is a primary problem, we label it a *phobic trait*. Marks (1970) has made a similar distinction for adult phobias. One rule to follow in differentiating between state and trait is to classify the condition as a phobic trait if the phobia is to be the primary treatment focus.

Two studies have used factor analysis to establish the basic dimensions of objects of children's fears. Scherer and Nakamura (1968) factored the responses of children to a fear inventory. Eight factors were obtained in an oblique rotation. Miller, Barrett, Hampe, and Noble (1972b) factored parents' ratings of

Table 1. Proposed Nosology for Child Phobia

I. Physical Injury	II. Natural Events	III. Social Anxiety	IV. Miscellaneous
A. Abstract	A. Storms	A. School	1. Dirt
1. War	1. Tornadoes, floods,	1. Young (Age 3-10)	2. Furry toys
2. Riots	earthquakes	(a) Type I	3. Sirens
3. Poisoned food	2. Lightning	(b) Type II	4. People who are old
4. Specific foods	3. Thunder	2. Old (Age 11-22)	5. Crossing a street
5. Dying	B. Dark	(a) Type I	6. People who are ugly
6. Someone in family dying	C. Enclosed places	(b) Type II	7. Loud sounds, as caps, firecrackers,
7. Seeing someone wounded	1. Bathrooms	B. Separation	explosions
8. Being wounded	2. Closets	1. Separation from parents	8. People in uniforms, a policeman,
9. Someone in family getting	3. Elevators	2. Parts of house	mailmen, etc.
ill	4. Confined or locked up	3. Going to sleep at night	9. People of the opposite sex
10. Becoming ill	5. Strange rooms	C. Performance	10. Having bowel movements
11. Germs	D. Animals	1. Tests or examinations	11. Members of another race
12. Choking	1. Snakes	2. Being criticized	
13. Having an operation	2. Insects, spiders	3. Making mistakes	
14. Hospitals	3. Rats or mice	4. Reciting in class	
15. Hell	4. Frogs or lizards	D. Social Interactions	
16. The devil	5. Dogs or cats	1. Attending social events	
17. Breaking a religious law	6. Horses or cows	2. Making another person	
18. Being kidnapped	E. Other	angry	
19. Getting lost	1. Fire	3. Crowds	
20. Being adopted	2. Frightening thoughts or	4. Being touched by others	
21. Parents getting a divorce	daydreams	E. Medical Procedures	
22. Going crazy	3. Ghosts	1. Doctors or dentists	
B. Concrete	4. Being alone	2. Getting a shot	
1. Flying in airplane	5. Nightmares	F. Other	
2. High places	6. Space creatures or monsters	1. Riding in a car or	
3. Deep water	7. Faces at window	bus	
4. Strangers	8. Masks or puppets		
5. Being seen naked	9. Sight of blood		
	10. People with deformities		
	11. Toilets		

92

children's fears and obtained three factors using a varimax rotation. The first factor in the Miller et al. study described fear of physical injury based on societal or man-made dangers such as wars, kidnapping, and food poisoning. The second factor described fears of natural events, such as storms and the dark. The central threat seemed to be the child's inability to live comfortably on his own with nature. The third factor indicated psychic and social stress; fears of examination, school, social events, being criticized, and being separated from parents.

Upon comparing Scherer and Nakamura's results with our work, we decided that their eight factors could be reduced to our three dimensions. Since neither of these studies has been cross-validated, and since Lapousse and Monk (1959) report major differences between parent and child perceptions of fear, it would be premature to advance more than a tentative scheme at this point. On the other hand, both studies indicate that fear tends to cluster around particular sets of objects. This tendency suggests an underlying dimensionality, which, in turn, suggests that phobic objects do not occur randomly, but many are interrelated. For a given patient, treatment of one phobia within a dimension should reduce the aversiveness connected with other stimuli within that dimension. In addition, if factor analysis yields anything more than just phenotypes, the same treatment should be applicable to all phobics within a given dimension. For these reasons, we decided to use the three primary factors of physical injury, natural events, and social anxiety as the major categories of child phobia.

We have placed the 81 items of the Louisville Fear Survey (Miller et al., 1972b) within the scheme according to their factor loadings with a few exceptions. We have subdivided physical injury into concrete and abstract objects. This distinction is not only self-evident, but it may have treatment implications insofar as concrete objects can be made available for *in vivo* therapy while abstract objects must be dealt with conceptually. Marks (1970) has found that the prognosis for adult animal-phobics is better than for all other phobics. This may possibly be true of all phobias of concrete objects.

Natural Events has been divided into five sub-categories; Storms, Dark, Enclosed Spaces, Animals, and Other. The reason for this is based upon treatment and assessment strategies. We do not know if treatment of storm phobias would be any different from treatment of fears of the dark, but if *in vivo* therapy or assessments are to be made, the groupings have considerable utility. Most clinical facilities, for example, have dark rooms and enclosed spaces available for *in vivo* therapy or assessment, and could easily house small animals. *In vivo* tests of storms, on the other hand, would have to be made with "sight and sound" effects or field observations. Thus this grouping is made with an eye toward *in vivo* therapy and assessment of therapeutic effects. When prognostic and differential treatment effects are known, these would be incorporated into the scheme.

Social Anxiety is divided into six sub-categories: School, Separation, Performance, Social Interactions, Medical Procedures, and Other. Placing School under Social Anxiety was arbitrary, since much evidence suggests a separate classification would be more appropriate. For example, females loaded significantly on this factor $(r = .63)$, but males did not $(r = .17)$. In another study, we found that School Phobia correlated only .26 on the fear scale of the Louisville Behavior Check List, which suggested that a School Phobia was different from other phobias (Miller, Barrett, Hampe, & Noble, 1971b). These correlations, as well as clinical experience, suggest that fear of school can be due to causes other than social stress. Stimuli such as storms, riding a bus, or separation anxiety may elicit a fear of school. However, we believe that for most school phobics, the primary problem is social anxiety. Therefore, we have placed this disorder under Category 3.

The major prognostic variable found in our own work, as well as in the literature on school phobia, is the age of the child. In our study, 96% of the children under 10 years of age who received treatment were free of their phobia within 14 weeks, while only 45% of those 11 and older were symptom-free. This is the general trend in the literature (Coolidge et al. 1960; Eisenberg, 1958; Smith, 1970), but there are exceptions (Gittelman-Klein & Klein, 1971; Hersov, 1960a). We believe that future studies will show that age is the primary prognostic variable in school phobia, and thus have included it within our scheme. We have not included age under the other phobic types, since we could find no studies bearing on the question.

Types I and II School Phobics refer to a distinction made first by Coolidge, Hahn, and Peck (1957), and refined by Kennedy (1965). We have dropped Kennedy's grade distinction, since we have found age to be such an important variable. Table 2 provides the characteristics of Types I and II. Six of nine items is sufficient to make a differential diagnosis.

At this point the literature is unclear as to the relationship of age and type of school phobia. We believe the primary variable is age, but there will be some young Type II's and some old Type I's. Studies are needed to determine the additional contribution provided by the breakdown of Types I and II. The only study we located was Weiss and Burke (1970), who found young Type II's responded well to hospitalization. They believed that outpatient treatment would have been difficult, but it was not tried, so we do not know.

The remainder of Category III is broken into content areas for which significance is yet to be established. One problem concerns overlapping classifications within Category III. For example, many authors argue that school phobia is basically a separation problem. We classed a child as a separation problem when there was evidence of problems of separation in areas of the child's life other than that of school. If, however, the child would leave his home and parents to visit friends or relatives, but would not go to school, we considered the child school-phobic. Another classification problem arises when a child has a specific

Table 2.   Characteristics of Types I and II School Phobics

Type I	Type II
1. The present illness is the first episode.	1. Second, third, or fourth episode.
2. Monday onset, following an illness the previous Thursday or Friday.	2. Monday onset following minor illness not a prevalent antecedent.
3. An acute onset.	3. Incipient onset.
4. Expressed concern about death.	4. Death theme not present.
5. Mother's physical health in question; actually ill or child thinks so.	5. Health of mother not an issue.
6. Good communication between parents.	6. Poor communication between parents.
7. Mother and father well adjusted in most areas.	7. Mother shows neurotic behavior; father, a character disorder.
8. Father competitive with mother in household management.	8. Father shows little interest in household or children.
9. Parents achieve understanding of dynamics easily.	9. Parents very difficult to work with.

fear within school, such as being called upon to recite in a particular class. In such cases, even though the child refuses to go to school, we believe that a recitation phobia is a more accurate diagnosis.

Finally, a list of items on which we have no information is included under Miscellaneous. Hopefully, as evidence accumulates, all items can be placed within the three major categories.

This scheme only partially meets our criteria. School Phobia is further classified to indicate prognosis and perhaps treatment strategy. The younger school-phobic has a much better prognosis than the older, and hospitalization may be necessary for Type II School-Phobics, while short-term management therapy may be all that is necessary for the young Type I School-Phobic. At the moment, these are tentative conclusions from the literature, and rigorous research is needed to affirm these hypotheses. Despite these limitations, the scheme clearly delineates the questions that need answering for school phobia. For other phobias the scheme is based on conventional wisdom and our factor analysis. The age and type breakdown of school-phobics may be very useful for all phobics, but this is not yet known. The breakdowns included in the scheme have advantages only for treatment planning and evaluation. None of the categories have the advantage of research behind them. Nothing is known, for example about when fears of the dark should be treated, nor is it known how best to treat them. Neither is it clear that fear of the dark is a unitary phenomenon. There may be many reasons why children fear the dark, and treatment may best be based upon those diverse reasons. The main point is that the categories should be functional, and only research can determine whether the categories suggested in this scheme have utility for prognosis, treatment, or assessment. We hope that eventually, the scheme could incorporate such information.

ASSESSMENT

Determining the presence and intensity of a phobia is a difficult undertaking if one goes beyond a verbal report. The classical literature on phobia is misleading because it gives the impression that a phobia is such an obvious phenomenon that measurement is unnecessary. Thus when Freud (1962) studied Little Hans, it apparently did not occur to him to determine whether the child was, in fact, afraid of horses. Acceptance of a parent's report is suspect in view of the Lapousse and Monk (1959) evidence that mothers report 41% fewer fears for their children than do the children themselves. More significant is the Jersild and Holmes (1935) finding that a fear stimulus is often quite complex. A child, for example, may be afraid of the dark only when alone. He may not be afraid of being alone during the day nor in the dark when with someone else. It is the combination of aloneness and dark that evokes the fear. This problem of stimulus complexity is also illustrated by the fact that Jersild and Holmes found, in an experimental situation, that a small energetic dog evoked more fear than a large, lethargic one. This suggests that energy level is a more important variable than size in children's fear of dogs. Also, we found (Miller et al., 1972b) that phobias were often unpredictable, that monophobias were rare, and that phobic stimuli were complex. This is consistent with the finding by Lang (1966) in adult phobics of a positive, but low correlation of subjective reports of phobia, behavior ratings, and physiological measurements. These observations all point to the fact that phobias are often variable responses to multiple stimuli and that assessment of phobia is a complex problem. Reliability and validity are as difficult to establish in phobics as in other manifestations of psychopathology. Thus it is important to discuss ways in which investigators have attempted to measure and evaluate child phobias.

Phobias are expressed through three modalities: behavior, subjective experience, and physiological responses. Direct observation of phobic behavior can be made in the laboratory when the controlling stimulus is available for presentation. Such a situational test was first reported by Watson (1921) in his study of infant startle responses. Since then, other investigators have employed similar techniques. Holmes (Jersild & Holmes, 1935) studied children experimentally from ages two to six using the following stimuli: Being left alone, noise, a falling board, the dark, a stranger, walking on a high board, a snake, and a large dog. Interest in situational tests was renewed by Lang's (1963) work with snakes. His model uses a room containing a box in which a large snake is placed. Floor stripes placed one foot apart extend from the door to the snake. The subject is asked to enter the room and to go as close to the snake as possible. The distance between the farthest approach and the snake becomes a quantitative measure of the phobia. Many studies with adults, but only a few with children, have used the situational test. The work of Bandura et al. (1967) with children who feared dogs is a notable exception.

When the phobic stimulus is not available for direct laboratory study, behavior can be evaluated in the field by trained or nontrained observers such as parents or teachers. Such observations are often the only alternative to the child's report of his phobic behavior. Only parents, or a participant observer can observe bedtime behaviors, reaction to certain foods, illnesses in the family, and such. Teachers are the obvious observers of behavior on tests or while speaking in front of the class. Trained field observers are generally more reliable than either parents or teachers, but they are expensive and alter the situation which they are observing. Also, Patterson et al. (1968) reported that even highly trained observers tend to be affected by the situation they are observing, so that within a month of field observations, correlations between observers drop from the mid-90s to mid-60s. Thus observers, whether they be parents, teachers, or participant observers, who record observations of children's behavior directly require training and frequent retraining to ensure collection of good data. Fortunately, Patterson (1968) and Caldwell and Honig (1971) provided some of the complex technology needed in such efforts.

When direct observations are not available, indirect methods have to be used. Retrospective ratings of fear behavior are probably even less reliable than concurrent observations, but they are quicker and less expensive to obtain. In our study of phobia we had parents rate the intensity and extensity, (extensity meaning the extent to which the fear affected the child's life), on a 7-point scale. The geometric mean of these ratings was used as an indication of the severity of a given phobia. We found that parents tended to overestimate severity at intake, but that in time parents' and clinicians' ratings were highly correlated. This suggests that ratings could be used as a criterion measure for follow-up. In addition to ratings of specific fears, two inventories are available: Scherer and Nakamura (1968) and Miller et al., (1972b). For school anxiety Sarason et al. (1953) have developed quite an extensive inventory, and Castaneda, McCandless, and Palermo (1956) have adapted the Taylor Manifest Anxiety Scale for children. A fear scale, consisting of parent ratings, is available in the Louisville Behavior Check List which provides an overall fear index in relation to other types of deviant behaviors (Miller et al., 1971b). Miller (1972) has developed an anxiety scale for the School Behavior Check List that provides evidence of fear behavior in the school. Berg and McGuire (1971) used the Highlands Dependency Inventory to study the extent of dependent behavior in school phobias. All of these inventories are useful for some purposes, and all are subject to the problems inherent in ratings.

Perhaps the most widely used method for obtaining indirect information is the interview. The interview has been studied extensively as an information source, and many biases and distortions are known to occur. Despite these limitations, the interview remains the central clinical tool, probably because a relationship is being built and maintained while information is gathered.

To illustrate how the interview is used to gain information, as well as how the interviewer's theoretical orientation shapes the information obtained, we quote from two case studies.

Smith and Sharpe (1970) noted that a standard interviewing technique failed to identify the stimuli associated with a 13-year-old boy's school phobia. Using a behaviorally oriented technique, they asked him to visualize and minutely describe a school day. They noted at which stages of his description behavioral indications of anxiety occurred. These indications included flushing of skin, increased body movements, vocal tremors, and muscular tension. This procedure indicated that he became highly anxious at the prospect of being called on to speak in mathematics or literature class and of having to answer teachers' questions. Neither visualization of home or his mother evoked manifest anxiety. Here the use of visual imagery and nonverbal cues helped to clarify the noxious stimuli. This information was then used to set up a hierarchy for implosive therapy, which in this instance was successful.

Mellita Sperling (1961), beginning from a psychoanalytic frame of reference, discussed a case of a 12-year-old female, whose school phobia began when she became upset with a teacher who took her music book away in class. Instead of eating lunch at school that day, she went home and found her mother gone. Upon telephoning her father, she learned that her mother had gone to the doctor to get an allergy shot. Next morning, the child did not feel well, but went to school.

For several days, the child was upset until one day she became panicky and her mother had to go to school and take her home. The mother was asked if the patient had any reason to be concerned about her visit to the doctor. The mother related that on the Sunday before the first incident in school, she had fainted during a church ceremony while sitting next to the child. The mother had also fainted 5 years before in her presence due to a gall bladder disease for which she received an injection and an operation. When the child was interviewed, she described the story of the music teacher and going home to find her mother missing; she did not relate the previous history. The child was reminded of the earlier fainting episode, which she remembered:

I suggested to her that her mother's recent fainting had brought back fears which she must have had when her mother fainted and was operated upon . . . without realizing it she had been worried about her mother since the incident in church, and that she came home for lunch because the incident in school had in some way increased her worry . . . not finding mother home and then learning that she was at the doctor's office had intensified and confirmed her fear about mother being in danger, a fear of which she had not been consciously aware. I told her that children sometimes have angry feelings toward their mothers, and, because they also believe in the magic power of their thoughts, they are afraid that something terrible may happen to mother. I assured her that thoughts and wishes are not dangerous and cannot kill anyone, but added that such thoughts can cause much fear in the child who has them and does not want to acknowledge them . . . I pointed out that this was really a conflict within herself which had to do with her feelings about mother and not a conflict with the teacher at school . . . my patient, too, went back to school the day after her interview [pp. 510–511].

These two cases illustrate how different frames of reference shape the inquiry process to elicit information necessary to fulfill the applied aspect of the theory. Smith and Sharpe needed information on the stimuli currently arousing anxiety to implode the child, while Sperling wanted information to clarify the preconscious conflict which could then be made conscious. Each approach adds to the interviewing process a dimension that should be considered when attempting to understand a child's phobia.

It is also possible to assess phobia through subjective measurements of fear made by the person who experiences it. One may rate the intensity of his feelings either in the presence of the stimulus or from his memory of past events. Such ratings can be made on single fears or on an inventory of fears. The inventories give an estimate of the total amount of focalized anxiety experienced by the person. However, children's subjective reports are difficult to appraise. We found some children who seemed to glory in describing their fears, while other children were very reticent. Some even refused to communicate at all. One child objected strongly to using fear as an explanation of his refusal to attend school. He simply maintained that he did not like school. We suspected that fear was a very unpleasant word for him to associate with himself. Thus subjective ratings pose very special problems when obtained from children, especially young children. Walk (1956) reports a method for obtaining subjective reports of fear by asking the subject to estimate his anxiety on a fear thermometer in which zero (0) represents no fear and the top of the scale represents extreme fear. We used a fear thermometer with children, but did not analyze the data, since our clinical observer thought that many of the estimates were random guesses by children. We have come to believe that the interview allows an adult to judge the child's emotional responses, which, when added to all other data, provide important qualitative information about the phobia. However, we question the value of a quantified estimate of subjective fears by children as an independent estimate of phobia. Much research needs to be done in this area before confidence can be placed in children's subjective reports.

Physiological measures of anxiety have an extensive research history and can be obtained from most autonomic channels; blood pressure, heart rate, muscular tension, or sweating. Instruments are available for obtaining measures of autonomic responses when the subject is presented with the phobic stimulus or its verbal equivalent.

A number of investigators have studied the psychophysiological aspects of adult phobias (Lacey, 1958; Leitenberg, Agras, Butz, & Winzce, 1971; Lader, 1967; Wilson, 1966; Marks, 1969; Lang, 1970), but we have found little work on children. This is, perhaps, a promising area but technical and equipment problems are so enormous that this must be considered a highly specialized and complex area of research. The primary problem lies in the well-established fact that each individual has his own idiosyncratic way of reacting to stress so that intragroup measures are difficult to establish. For the moment, then, physiological measures of childhood phobia are promising tools of the future, but have little clinical use.

It should be noted in this discussion that two critical assessment issues have not been considered. The first is the psychoanalytic contention that phobias are external representations of internal conflicts. Melitta Sperling's (1961) case reported above illustrates that the distinction between fear and phobia is that phobias represent unconscious conflicts and diminution of phobias is impossible without a resolution of the conflict:

No matter how difficult the cases may appear clinically, the basic conflict underlying the symptoms is the same and the phobia demands prompt treatment based on psychoanalytic understanding. . . . The precipitating events that touch off the acute anxiety, manifested in school phobia, are always events that unconsciously are interpreted by the child as a danger to his mother's life and his own life . . . a phobia is not amenable to reason, persuasion, or punishment. . . . I also do not believe in "self cures" of phobics. . . . I recommend . . . exposing to the patient as soon as possible the basic conflict underlying the phobia [pp. 507–508].

Psychoanalysts have studied phobias too extensively for us to brush aside their contention; yet we see no way to assess unconscious conflicts. Case examples (Arieti, 1961; Bornstein, 1935; Freud, 1962; Renik, 1972; Sperling, 1961; Waugh, 1967) of child phobias are subject to so many divergent interpretations (Rachman & Costello, 1961; Wolpe & Rachman, 1960) that answers are not forthcoming. Therefore, until measurements of unconscious conflicts can be made, we have chosen to table the analytic contention and to assess phobias in terms of behavioral, subjective, and physiological components.

The second assessment issue concerns the distinction in behavior theory between respondent and operant conditioning. In theory, phobias arising from respondent conditioning should be reduced through extinction while contingency management would be necessary for operant phobias. We find this an impossible distinction to make with child phobias, and point out that Mowrer would have predicted our difficulty. But if we accept the respondent-operant distinction, clinical histories often point to both types of conditioning. Furthermore, phobias are so commanding once they emerge that reinforcement schedules are always established within the family. It is then impossible to determine with current methods whether observed reinforcements are simply maintaining the phobia or whether they played a part in its etiology. In brief, we find the distinction between operant and respondent conditioning to be of little practical value. Therefore, we have omitted the distinction both in the definition and in the assessment procedures.

There are advantages and disadvantages associated with measurements from each expressive modality. Direct behavior ratings have the advantage of reliable quantification and of openness to multiple observers. This is particularly true when the phobic stimulus is presented in an experimental situation where the measure is a function of the subject's approach behavior. Laboratory control can only occur, however, with a limited number of simple and concrete phobic objects, and has the disadvantage of selecting only subjects who invariably respond with fear to the phobic stimulus. Such subjects probably may have little in common with phobics who present themselves in clinical situations. Also, direct behavior ratings do not elicit subjective feelings and do not distinguish low motivation from phobic discomfort. That is, failure to approach could reflect either immobilization or disinterest. For research on specific stimuli, however, direct behavior ratings are probably the most objective measure of phobic behavior.

Field observations have the advantage of access to the child's exposure to many stimuli that would otherwise go unobserved, but of course observer error is introduced. Parents and teachers are often "members of the problem," so that they do not give unbiased observations, but trained observers are very expensive and, as previously noted, are subject to the influence of the situation. Furthermore, we have found that phobic responses, even of long standing, often disappear during the process of evaluation. One example occurred when the authors observed a child with an elevator/escalator phobia make three unsuccessful attempts to ride the escalator before her mother got on and left her. At that moment another child stepped on the escalator and our patient watched his every move, imitated his behavior, and successfully rode away. She spent the rest of the morning riding both the escalator and elevator. The mother could not believe that this occurred because her child had previously made shopping an impossible undertaking. This case illustrates not only the effects of modeling, but also that our assessment procedures themselves seemed to have an effect. The situational test that we had come to observe actually served as a therapeutic procedure. We noted enough of these variable responses to become convinced that phobias, as reported by parents, are subject to many effects that can be sorted out only by time and extended case study.

In view of the complex problems associated with the assessment of phobia and the lack of consensus as to the best assessment method, we recommend an intensive clinical case study, followed by a rating of the phobia's intensity and extensity. After evaluating a number of procedures including field observers and situational tests, we concluded that clinical behavior ratings based on all material was the best indicator of phobia. To obtain these ratings, we interviewed the parents intensively to establish the child's specific fear reactions, as well as the context in which the event took place. In addition, we attempted to establish how much of the child's life span was affected by the phobia. Parents also completed the Louisville Behavior Check List (Miller et al., 1971a) so˙that we could determine whether there were other problem areas in the child's life, and the Louisville Fear Survey Schedule (Miller et al., 1972) to let us know if there were other fears. Generally, children did have other behavioral problems and phobias that were not reported in the interviews. The child was interviewed to obtain his views and reactions to his world and to his problems. In addition, when feasible, a situational test was run. Following these interviews, we checked with the mother for 5 days, by telephone, to establish frequency counts of fear reactions. This information was then presented at a case conference. When the child had multiple phobias, the most disabling of them was selected as the target phobia and then each conference participant rated the intensity and extensity of that phobia on a 7-point scale. The geometric mean was obtained for each rating, and the mean of all ratings became a measure of the severity of the phobia. We accepted into treatment children whose phobias were rated 3.0 or higher. If we carefully explained these rating procedures to parents after the initial assessment, we found that succeeding parent ratings and staff ratings agreed very well. Thus parent ratings were used in follow-up evaluations.

To recapitulate, phobias are seldom invariant responses to simple, discrete stimuli. Rather, phobic responses range from highly variable and episodic to invariant, while phobic stimuli range from simple to complex. There are instances of monophobias, but these are rare, for generally a child has several stimuli that elicit his anxiety. In the case of multiple phobias, a single target phobia must be selected for a treatment focus. Factor analysis suggests that the multiple-phobic stimuli are organized into dimensions which perhaps reflect response gradients so that reduction of anxiety associated with one stimulus would be followed by a reduction of anxiety toward all stimuli in that dimension. We prefer an intense clinical case study to assess phobias except in instances where an investigator needs a homogenous population to study the approach behavior to simple phobic stimuli. In this case, the situational test would be appropriate.

CHARACTERISTICS OF CHILD PHOBIA

Age of Onset

Freud believed that the prototypical trauma for all anxiety was the birth experience followed by separation anxiety as the infant became aware of his individual existence. Examining the question empirically, Watson and Rayner (1920) postulated that just two situations evoked a fear response in the newborn; a loud sound and a loss of support. Later, investigations by Irwin (1932) and Shirley (1933) raised doubts as to the universality of Watson's two factors. Other investigators were able to show the effect of maturation on fear. For example, Jones and Jones (1928) found that children up to two years of age showed no fear of a large harmless snake, while children aged three were cautious, and by age four definite signs of fear were displayed, and in adults were more pronounced. It is now generally recognized that fear and anxiety arise as a normal consequence of social development (Levitt, 1967), and result from the interaction between maturation and personal experience. While many fears are age-specific and tend to be resolved as the child matures, others are atypical for a given age, either arising from individual experiences or lingering far past the appropriate age. To diagnose a phobia then, it is necessary to distinguish age-appropriate from inappropriate fears. Empirical data are sketchy, but the major outlines of the effects of age on fear are available.

Fear does not appear to be a significant variable during the first six months of life, although loud noises and loss of support can evoke fear in some newborns. Somewhere between the sixth and ninth month, the child begins to develop an awareness of strangers, becoming frightened when given over to nonfamiliar caretakers. Fear of strangers evolves into a more general separation anxiety which is usually evoked when the mother leaves the child with someone else, but is also shown when the child refuses to leave the mother to explore the world on his own. Separation anxiety usually reaches its most acute phase at the end of the second year of life for most children, and is usually mastered by the fourth year of life. Many authorities believe that when mastery does not occur, separation anxiety becomes the core problem in school phobia (Rodriguez, Eisenberg, & Rodriguez, 1959; Johnson, Falstein, Szurek, & Svendsen, 1941; Eisenberg, 1958). Around age two, when toilet training begins for most children, fear of the toilet is not uncommon. Fears of imaginary creatures, death, robbers, and being alone begin around 15 months of age and tend to increase up to age four, and then show a steady decrease until age 11 when there is again an upsurge of fear (MacFarlane, Allen, & Honzik, 1954). Dogs are the predominant fear at age three, while by the fourth year the fear of the dark predominates. At age six, fear of school becomes a problem and declines in frequency until age 11 when there is an acceleration of school-associated anxiety (Smith, 1970). By age 12, there appears to be a decrease in fears of natural events and at some point between age 12 and adulthood a cluster of fears centering around sexuality, abortion, suicide, defective children, and such, emerge. Fears of injury and social anxieties stay throughout the life span from the time they originate in early childhood. Table 3 gives the dominant fears arising or being maintained at each age level. It is clear from this survey that many fears are age-related and will dissipate as the child matures and gains a greater understanding of his world. In our definition of phobia, we excluded such age-related fears. Thus phobias are exaggerated developmental fears, or a continuation of such fears past their expected decay point, or fears of stimuli other than those associated with the developmental period.

Table 3.   Developmental Fears at Different Age Levels

Age	Fears
0-6 Months	Loud noises, loss of support
6-9 Months	Strangers
1st Year	Separation, injury, toilet
2nd Year	Imaginary creatures, death, robbers
3rd Year	Dogs, being alone
4th Year	Dark
6-12 Years	School, injury, natural events, social
13-18 Years	Injury, social
19+ Years	Injury, natural events, sexual

Frequency

In this section, we examine the overall frequency of fear to be expected in the general population. Jersild and Holmes (1935) noted that children aged two to six had an average of 4.64 fears per child and manifested fear once every four and one half days. They concluded that overt fears were relatively infrequent at this age compared to other types of deviant behavior. Hagman (1932) found in a comparable group of children that there was an average of 2.7 fears per child. MacFarlane et al. (1954) reported that at least 90% of the children in their study had a specific fear at least once during the first 14 years of their lives and that up until the age of 12 at least 35% showed some fear. Lapousse and Monk (1959), in a general population sample of 482 children aged six to 12, found that 43% had seven or more fears and worries. They concluded that fears are quite common in children of this age. Each of these studies differs in the method of establishing and rating fears and each sampled from different sections of the country, so that findings are not absolutely comparable. However, it would appear that children aged two to six have about three fears on the average, and that 40% of the children aged six to 12 show some fears, perhaps as many as seven.

In a recent study of a general population sample of 249 children aged seven to 12, using the Louisville Fear Survey Schedule, the authors found that the number of excessive reactions were few. Moreover, while some stimuli evoked considerable fear, the child's family felt such strong reactions were normal. Table 4 shows parent rating of the percentage of fears at three intensity levels: no fear, normal or expected fear, and excessive or unrealistic fear. With a few exceptions, stimuli evoke extreme fear in less than 5% of the general population. The most typical response pattern approximates a J-curve in which 84% or more of the children show no fear of the stimuli, while 5 to 15% show what parents consider to be normal fear and 0 to 5% show excessive fears. Stimuli eliciting the J-curve pattern include dirt, furry toys, masks or puppets, old people, and toilets, as well as many others. Responses to a smaller group of stimuli more closely approximate a normal curve, in which 25 to 45% show no fear, 50 to 60% show normal fear, and 4 to 6% show excessive fear. This group includes snakes, rats, lightning, fire, and tornadoes, along with being wounded, getting shots, or being seen naked. The third group falls somewhere in between the first two with an approximately equal split between no fear and normal fear. This group includes stimuli such as insects, sight of blood, dark, ghosts, and war, along with being locked up, being kidnapped and many more. These different reaction patterns suggest that extreme fears (phobias) are rare in the seven to 12 age group. Fear behavior is observed quite frequently by parents, but it is considered normal. Also, Table 4 indicates that the intensity and frequency of fear reactions are a function of the stimulus object.

Table 4 also shows that snakes evoked the most extreme fear in girls in this age group (13%), followed by rats and mice (11%), and then by dark (8%), war (8%), and being kidnapped (8%), and being seen naked (8%). Boys, on the other hand, showed less overall fear than girls and reacted most to criticism (7%) and shots (7%), followed by snakes (6%) and deep water (5%). In our study of child phobia (Miller et al., 1972b) we found that 69% of our referrals were for school phobia which occurred in less than 1% of the general population. The next highest referral was for sleeping alone (9%) which occurs in 1% of the boys in the general population and in 2% of the girls. The third referral fear was of the dark (6%) which approximates the percentage found in the general population ($M = 3\%, F = 8\%$). However, quite a number of other fears occurred as frequently as fear of the dark which were not referred for treatment: snakes, rats/mice, death, deep water, tornadoes, space creatures, and war, and being seen naked, being criticized and being kidnapped. This suggests that the existence of excessive fear is not by itself cause for referral. The fear of school has such major secondary effects that even though it is rare, help is sought when it occurs. Fears of the dark and sleeping alone probably are sufficiently noxious to parents to cause them to seek help. We can postulate then, that as long as a child's excessive fear does not seriously impede the socialization process or interfere with the parents' lives, the children's phobias will not be brought to the attention of health professionals. When fears are merely passing episodes in the developmental process, their neglect is of no consequence, but when they represent a stable condition, they can cause considerable distress throughout the life span.

Prognosis and Natural History

Data on age-related fears do not reflect changes that take place over time for individual subjects. Hagman (1932), for example, found that 6% of the fears noted in his study disappeared within one week, 54% were gone in three months, and 100% had disappeared in three years.

Table 4. Frequency of Fears at Three Intensity Levels[a] in a General Population of 123 Boys and 126 Girls Between the Ages of Seven to 12

Fears	Male 1	Male 2	Male 3	Female 1	Female 2	Female 3
1. Dirt	93	7	0	86	14	0
2. Furry toys	98	2	0	98	2	0
3. Masks/puppets	95	5	0	90	10	0
4. Sirens	87	13	0	69	30	1
5. Insects or spiders	53	45	2	14	81	5
6. Frogs or lizards	72	28	0	24	71	5
7. Horses/cows	85	15	0	71	29	0
8. Dogs/cats	86	12	2	79	20	1
9. Snakes	28	66	6	5	82	13
10. Rats/mice	46	52	2	11	78	11
11. Storms	53	44	3	33	63	4
12. Lightning	46	51	3	24	73	3
13. Thunder	55	43	2	30	66	4
14. Fire	39	59	2	17	79	4
15. Old people	95	5	0	87	12	1
16. Crossing street	84	16	0	71	29	0
17. Sight of blood	57	41	2	40	57	3
18. People who are ugly	84	16	0	82	17	1
19. Faces at windows	56	42	2	38	57	5
20. Being kidnapped	55	43	2	38	54	8
21. Specific foods	90	10	0	79	20	1
22. Being alone	63	36	1	40	56	4
23. Being criticized	51	42	7	39	57	4
24. Being in the dark	51	46	3	34	58	8
25. Crowds	89	11	0	83	17	0
26. Strangers	60	39	1	45	53	2
27. Hospitals	57	41	2	60	39	1
28. Bathrooms	95	5	0	91	9	0
29. Closets	94	6	0	77	22	1
30. Toilets	96	4	0	91	9	0
31. Ghosts	51	46	3	38	59	3
32. The devil	54	44	2	34	63	3
33. Hell	53	45	2	39	56	5
34. School	93	6	1	90	10	0
35. Germs	77	22	1	67	32	1
36. Choking	67	32	1	61	37	2
37. Nightmares	63	35	2	54	40	6
38. Riots	63	36	1	54	44	2
39. Dying	54	45	1	48	49	3
40. Deep water	56	39	5	40	53	7
41. Tornadoes, floods, earthquakes	40	56	4	29	65	6
42. Space creatures, monsters	57	39	4	41	54	5
43. Food that might be poisoned	56	42	2	49	47	4
44. Riding in bus or car	93	7	0	87	13	0
45. Flying in airplane	73	26	1	60	38	2
46. Loud sounds, as caps, firecrackers, explosions	76	24	0	50	48	2
47. Being separated from parents	67	32	1	44	52	4
48. Parents getting divorce	76	21	3	62	33	5

106

Table 4 (Continued)

Fears	Male 1	Male 2	Male 3	Female 1	Female 2	Female 3
49. Reciting in class	58	41	1	45	52	3
50. Attending social events due to worries of rejection	76	23	1	71	29	0
51. Breaking religious law (sin)	57	41	2	51	48	1
52. War, enemy invasion bombing	52	45	3	51	41	8
53. Making another person angry	52	46	2	53	47	0
54. Entering a strange room	65	34	1	56	43	1
55. Being confined or locked up	49	50	1	37	56	7
56. Going to sleep at night	88	11	1	84	14	2
57. Being touched by others	89	11	0	78	22	0
58. People with deformities	74	26	0	59	40	1
59. Uniformed people policemen, etc.	90	10	0	83	15	2
60. High places	61	35	4	53	44	3
61. Opposite sex	90	9	1	85	15	0
62. Enclosed places	77	23	0	63	35	2
63. Elevators	89	11	0	78	20	2
64. Certain part of house (attic, etc.)	83	15	2	68	31	1

Fears	Male 1	Male 2	Male 3	Female 1	Female 2	Female 3
65. Being ill	67	32	1	63	36	1
66. Family member becoming ill	61	37	2	55	44	1
67. Going crazy (insane)	80	18	2	79	20	1
68. Getting lost	57	41	2	51	47	2
69. Seeing someone wounded	29	67	4	24	72	4
70. Being wounded	29	68	3	29	67	4
71. Being seen naked	38	59	3	26	66	8
72. Having bowel movements	92	7	1	89	10	1
73. Receiving shots	36	57	7	33	64	3
74. Doctors or dentists	49	48	3	38	60	2
75. Having operation	38	60	2	39	56	5
76. Family member dying	45	51	4	37	56	7
77. Members of another race	85	15	0	76	22	2
78. Making mistakes, doing something wrong	44	53	3	37	60	3
79. Frightening thoughts or daydreams	76	24	0	69	29	2
80. Tests, examinations	58	41	1	41	57	2
81. Being adopted	84	14	2	73	23	4

[a] Intensity levels: 1. no fear observed; 2. normal or reasonable fear; 3. unreasonable or excessive fear.

107

In an interesting study in Japan, Abe (1972) had mothers of three-year-olds describe their fears and the fears of their children. He also asked the maternal grandmothers to describe the fears the mothers had at age three. He found that the mothers' current phobias dated from their childhood, but that 65% of the mothers who had phobias as children had no symptoms in adult life. Marks partially confirmed Abe's findings in his retrospective study of adult phobics (1971). He found animal phobias tended to arise in early childhood, while most situational and social phobias began after puberty. Agoraphobia began at all ages, but the peak onset age was adolescence.

Hellman (1962) gives a clinical description of the dissipation of child phobias described by Abe. A 2½-year-old female child developed an acute and overwhelming separation reaction when she was left on the spur of the moment by her mother at the Hampstead Nursery during World War II. At first, there was continuous and incessant crying, followed by gradual and almost complete social withdrawal and loss of interaction with surroundings. She made and maintained an extremely close and exclusive relationship with her nurse to whom she clung with desperation. This condition lasted for six months before it began to abate. As an adult, a follow-up study revealed an extroverted, competent person with a satisfactory career, and good social relationships and opportunities for gratification in work and leisure. Hellman noted that she had survived the separation trauma with less negative effect than expected by the original caretakers and predicted by analytic theory. Hampe et al. (1973) found that when 62 phobic children six to 15 years old were followed up two years after termination of treatment, only 7% still had a severe phobia, and 80% were symptom free. Bandura, Grusec, and Menlov (1967) found that untreated children with a fear of dogs did not improve over a one-week period, while treated children lost their fear. Agras (1972) found in a five-year follow-up of 30 phobics that 100% of persons under 20 were free of their symptoms, while only 43% of the adults had shown significant improvement and 37% were worse.

A number of follow-up studies have been done with school phobias. Coolidge et al. (1964) followed up 56 children 10 years after initial intake. Fifty-four of the 56 children had returned to and remained in school, and two-thirds were performing up to IQ expectations. One of the two that did not return was psychotic. Most of the group were described as passive and compliant in their school behavior, having many problems in making friends, and being slow and cautious in their dating pattern. One third of the group were still experiencing moderate to serious difficulties. Hersov (1960), 12 months after termination of treatment, evaluated 50 school phobics, 28 of whom had been hospitalized, and found that 68% had returned to school. Recovery was not related to age, sex, IQ, duration of symptoms, or quality of family relationships. Rodriquez et al. (1959) followed up 41 cases of school phobia three years after termination of treatment and found that 71% were attending school regularly and that 89% of children below 11 years of age were free of fear as contrasted to 64% of children 11 years and older. Berg (1970) found that 59% of adolescent school phobics admitted to an in-patient service had recovered one year after discharge and 41% had not. Weiss and Burke (1970) found in a five to 10 year follow-up that 16 school-phobic children eight to 16 years old who were treated in a hospital had little problem returning to school after hospitalization. All but one graduated from high school and achieved up to IQ level. About one-half had good social adjustments, but one-half remained shy and hesitant to date and had few friends. With a few exceptions, all were found to maintain good performance at work and in school and were economically independent. The exceptions to these general findings were two boys, originally diagnosed as psychotic, who remained completely dependent and unproductive at follow-up.

Phobias in adults have a different history. Tucker (1956) followed up a group of 100 adult phobics and found that only 28% had recovered, 53% had improved, and 19% were unchanged. Marks (1971) found in a four-year follow-up that only 26% had much improved, 32% improved, and 42% showed no change. Glick (1970) reported a 37% success rate with 48 adult phobics. Errera and Coleman (1963) found at a 23-year follow-up of 19 adult phobics that 79% had remained essentially unchanged, while only 21% were improved. Contrary to these findings, Terhune (1949) reported that 67% of his 86 adult phobic patients recovered and 24% improved, while only 9% showed no change.

In summary, it appears that fears and phobias in children under 10 years of age arise and dissipate rapidly. In the Miller and Bandura studies this process was hastened with psychotherapy. There is little information on the natural history of phobias during adolescence, except for school phobia, which has a poorer prognosis during adolescence than during preadolescence. However, the long-range prognosis appears quite good for most adolescent school phobics unless they show psychotic symptoms. Phobia in adults appears to be much more intractable since full recovery is somewhere between 20 and 30%. The new behavior therapies hold promise, but firm evidence of therapeutic efficacy is far from clear at this writing.

Personality Characteristics

Many investigators attribute various types of personality characteristics to phobic children. Unfortunately, there is very little systematic research upon which to draw conclusions and much that is available is limited to school phobia. The best documentation in this area comes from studies using behavioral check lists for parent and teacher ratings of deviant behavior (Achenbach, 1966; Cattell & Coan, 1957; Dreger, Lewis, Rich, Miller, Reed, Overlade, Taffel, & Flemming, 1964; Miller, 1967, 1971a, 1971b; Peterson, 1961). Each of these studies has clearly shown that manifest anxiety is an independent dimension in child psychopathology. Miller (1967) showed that manifest anxiety was one aspect of a behavioral triad making up an inhibition dimension. The other two aspects were social withdrawal and sensitivity. That anxiety is an independent dimension has been confirmed by investigators using other methods. Lapousse and Monk (1959), for example, found no correlation between child fears and other forms of deviant behavior. Jersild and Holmes (1935) found a correlation of .58 between children's fears observed by parents and those observed in experimental situations. MacFarlane et al. (1954) found low correlations with irritability (r = .28) and temper (r = .21), but high correlation with the inhibition behaviors such as timidity (r = .64), overdependence (r = .35), and mood swings (r = .31). Scherer and Nakamura (1968) found a correlation of .49 between total number of fears and the children's manifest anxiety scale. This was affirmed by L'Abate (1960) for girls, but not for boys. L'Abate felt that different anxiety scales needed to be constructed for boys and girls. There is little doubt, then, that anxious behavior forms a specific dimension that can be recognized both at home and in school.

To what extent phobic children possess specific personality characteristics beyond the presenting behavior is still a moot question. Greenacre (1952) thought that anxious subjects had a predisposition to anxiety related to the prenatal or postnatal period of life that left an organic stamp on the child which heightened the anxiety potential. This tension in early infancy led to an increased and prolonged narcissism and later to an ineffective sense of reality. Leventhal and Sills (1967) have formulated this narcissistic characteristic in reference to school phobia. They noted that these children overvalue themselves and their achievements, and then try to hold onto their unrealistic self-image. When they are threatened in the school situation, they suffer anxiety and retreat to another situation where they can maintain their narcissistic self-image. Nichols (1970) attempted to test Leventhal's contention by comparing the self-concepts of school-phobics to other types of disturbed children, and found no support for Leventhal's thesis. We suspect that Leventhal did not formulate the proposition correctly and that Nichol's study is not an adequate test; but only further research can clarify this issue.

The Judge Baker group of investigators (Coolidge et al., 1960; Waldfogel et al., 1957) separated school phobias into two types, neurotic and characterological. The neurotic group tended to be younger, had acute and traumatic onset, and generally functioned well in other areas (Kennedy Type I). The characterological group were older and more disturbed. Symptoms in this second group had a more gradual onset, and were the culmination of a lengthy process. These children had a generalized fear of the outside world, were basically mistrusting, used projection and externalization, and refused to take responsibility for their feelings and actions. The central conflict in the characterological group revolved around the symbiotic relationship with the mother.

Other investigators believe the key conflict in school phobia to be separation anxiety. Johnson et al. (1941) were the first to suggest that the basic difficulty was in leaving home rather than in going to school. Eisenberg (1958) supported the contention and suggested that the problem was bilateral; that is, the involved parent (usually the mother) intensified and reciprocated the child's anxiety. Gittelman-Klein and Klein (1971), who found that children treated with imipramine returned to school, while a no-drug control group did not, challenged this argument. They argued that there could be no difference in reduction of communicated parental anxiety in the two groups, which separation theory would postulate, since each group received identical parental counseling. The difficulty with all of these ideas is that there is little systematic research and the one test of Leventhal's thesis was not adequate. Since there are common themes running through many of the clinical studies, we cannot discount the possibility of their validity, but as yet, we cannot draw any conclusions.

The available systematic studies on personality attributes of phobic children suggest that phobias, even school phobias, occur at all intelligence levels (Hampe et al., 1973; Hersov, 1960a, 1960b), although some studies with biased samples contradict this conclusion (Eisenberg, 1958). Miller et al. (1972b) also found that phobias in children were generally associated with an increase in many forms of deviant behavior as reported by parents and teachers although the primary increase was in inhibition.

Table 5 shows standard scores $(M = 50, SD = 10)$ at intake on the Louisville Behavior Check List, School Behavior Check List, and Louisville Fear Survey of 67 phobic children accepted for a psychotherapy project. It can be seen from Table 5 that all deviant scales were elevated above a matched general population sample except Aggression (Item 13) and Physical Injury (Item 18), while the nondeviant scales, Prosocial Behavior and Extraversion, were depressed. It appears that disturbance in one area tends to create disturbance in other areas.

Hersov (1960b) found that 74% of school phobics were timid and fearful away from home, but willful and dominating at home (e.g., Leventhal). He also found that 25% were passive and obedient at home. Hersov further found that as young children, school-phobics had had less experience in coping with parental absence, tended to be overprotected, and had high standards of work performance. Berg and McGuire (1971) also found school-phobics overly dependent shown by a high immaturity score and a low sociability score on the Highland Dependency Inventory.

In regard to mother–child relationships, Hersov (1960b) found that 50% of the mothers of school-phobics were overindulgent and dominated by the child, while 28% were demanding, severe, and overcontrolling. Fifty-four percent of the fathers were described as inadequate, passive, but good providers, while 28% were severe and dominating. Hersov (1960a) also noted a high incidence of neurosis in the families of school-phobic children.

These sketchy findings certainly point to no single type of personality or

Table 5. Scores on Louisville Behavior Check List, and Louisville Fear Survey at Intake on 67 Phobic Children Compared With Matched Sample of Children from the General Population

	Phobic		General		
	M	SD	M	SD	F^a
Louisville Behavior Check List					
1. Infantile aggression	60.95	15.01	49.11	7.77	31.43
2. Hyperactivity	57.30	13.14	49.20	8.19	17.48
3. Antisocial behavior	55.48	16.28	48.94	8.06	8.31
4. Social withdrawal	62.92	13.39	48.52	9.42	49.54
5. Sensitivity	64.63	17.12	49.50	9.78	37.65
6. Fear	73.08	21.22	49.91	7.67	67.50
7. Academic disability	55.14	10.97	49.63	10.98	8.08
8. Immaturity	58.75	15.10	49.17	9.63	18.31
9. Normal irritability	56.61	10.31	48.16	9.61	23.02
10. Rare deviance	1.84	1.45	0.08	0.27	91.72
11. Prosocial	43.09	14.54	55.27	14.08	23.14
School Behavior Check List					
12. Low need achievement	58.75	9.55	48.84	9.11	36.06
13. Aggression	54.14	11.49	51.44	10.37	1.95
14. Anxiety	71.52	13.59	49.59	10.07	107.48
15. Academic disability	51.93	10.18	48.28	8.67	4.78
16. Extraversion	39.73	15.52	49.31	11.28	15.94
Louisville Fear Survey for Children					
17. Natural events	57.49	14.47	47.28	9.60	22.57
18. Physical injury	48.94	11.17	47.31	9.26	0.80
19. Social stress	63.06	15.58	49.19	8.97	38.10

$^aF = 2.11, df = 19/108, p < .01.$

112

parent–child relationship that is associated with or that is specific to phobia. There is some indication that there are subtypes, the most frequent being the child who is inhibited outside the home, but who is a tyrant within the home. However, this is by no means the only pattern associated with phobia, and we have no idea how frequent such personalities and relationships develop with no consequent phobia. Also, this pattern has been noted in other forms of psychopathology. At this point, then, we must conclude that investigations have raised some interesting suppositions, but as yet there are no compelling answers.

THEORY

We stated at the beginning of this chapter that no adequate theory explains the etiology or the maintenance of phobia. Theories have been advanced, yet all fail to account for some aspects of the phenomenon. In this section, we discuss briefly the major theories which purport to account for phobia. Since our discussion of theory is sketchy, we urge readers to turn to original sources for a more comprehensive view of this complex subject.

There are two major theories and two minor but significant theories that compete for professional attention. Psychoanalytic theory was advanced in the early 1900s and became the dominant theory during the first half of the twentieth century. Behavior theory followed a few years later, but did not gain much support outside of the academic community until recently. Cognitive-developmental theory has contributed important insights, but no total explanation of phobia has been advanced by its adherents or by those advocating a transactional approach.

Sigmund Freud (1962) first formulated the psychoanalytic theory of phobia around the case of Little Hans. This theory has been altered and elaborated upon by Freud and other workers during the past 70 years (Arieti, 1961; Bornstein, 1935; Klein, 1945; Renik, 1972; Sperling, 1961; Waugh, 1967). Psychoanalytic theory proposes a structural hypothesis of personality which assumes three interacting groupings of function; the id, ego, and superego. When an instinctual impulse arises which clashes with realistic, self-preservative, or conscious-directed interests, a slight degree of anxiety is used as a signal to warn of impending danger. The anxiety signal mobilizes defensive maneuvers aimed at keeping the instinct under control, while simultaneously permitting the person to continue to function. Since the instinctual danger is internal and inescapable, externalization transfers the danger to an external object which then can be avoided, while displacement removes the danger from within the intimate family relationships to neutral objects, usually outside the home.

Freud believed that all phobias originated from libidinal (sexual) conflicts, but other theorists assumed that aggression and dependence also played an important role. Freud, however, distinguished different varieties of anxiety based upon the specific threat. Thus he explained the fear of the dark, of being left alone, and of strangers as deriving from the need for the presence of the mother. He postulated that libido was mobilized as tension increased (longing), and when discharge was not possible, "separation anxiety" occurred as a signal of danger of loss of mother. The next level of fear was of castration arising from the Oedipus conflict where the child's affection for the parent of the opposite sex created a fear of damage to the genitals because of the same-sex parent's jealousy. Superego anxiety, together with social anxiety, represented the next stage of anxiety development. What was formerly experienced as castration anxiety now became internalized as the disapproval of conscience. The ensuing guilt dominated the personality and regulated the person's actions. In brief, the conscious anxiety experienced by the person with a phobia was the result of unconscious anxiety produced by a conflict between id, ego, and superego. The unconscious anxiety was thus displaced to an external concrete object, which permitted the person to function except in the presence of the phobic object. The object was a symbol of the unconscious wish; thus by avoiding the object, one avoided expressing the forbidden wish.

Social learning theory has evolved as a strong competitor to psychoanalysis. While psychoanalytic theory was based primarily on clinical data, social learning theory emerged from the experimental laboratory. Within social learning, there are three divergent theories of behavior: Respondent Conditioning, Operant Conditioning, and the Two Factor Theory of Conditioning. Each of these assumes that phobias are learned. Respondent theory assumes that anxiety is the central aspect of the phobic behavior, and that any neutral stimulus that happens to make an impact on an individual at the time that a fear reaction occurs will subsequently evoke the fear reaction. If the original conditioning situation is of high intensity or if repeated some number of times, the conditioned fear will then tend to persist without obvious reinforcement. The phobic behavior persists paradoxically, since it is unpleasant. Having acquired an unpleasant association and reaction to a particular stimulus or situation, the person will tend to avoid exposure to this noxious stimulus. The tendency to avoid the noxious situation impedes spontaneous recovery, since learned patterns of behavior can only be extinguished by repeated nonreinforced behavior. Phobic responses are also subject to generalization so that the response may generalize to a range of stimuli similar to the original noxious stimulus. The essentials of the theory are summarized by Rachmann and Costello (1961, p. 101):

1. Phobias are learned responses.

2. Phobic stimuli, simple or complex, develop when they are associated temporally and spatially with a fear-producing state of affairs.

3. Neutral stimuli that are of relevance in the fear-producing situation and/ or make an impact on the person in the situation are more likely to develop phobic qualities than weak or irrelevant stimuli.

4. Repetition of the association between the fear situation and the new phobic stimuli will strengthen the phobia.

5. Associations between high-intensity fear situations and neutral stimuli are more likely to produce phobic reactions.

6. Generalization from the original phobic stimulus to stimuli of a similar nature will occur.

Operant theory postulates that behavior that is rewarded will tend to reoccur while behavior that is not rewarded will extinguish. This theory would assume that avoidance behavior observed in phobias, as well as many of the accompanying behaviors such as temper tantrums are positively and systematically reinforced. The primary reinforcers are social rewards dispensed by significant persons in the immediate environment, primarily members of the family. Attention, whether affectionate or punitive, seems to serve equally well as a reinforcer. Parents and other significant persons teach children to be afraid by selectively attending and rewarding fearful and avoidant behaviors. Thus children are taught fear of the dark, death, dogs, separation, school, and such, by parents' and age-mates' responding with affection, anger, or reassurance to the child's fear, cautious approaches, and avoidance of these situations. The child, in turn, learns that parents are sensitive to such behaviors and respond with much attention and preoccupation so that a little fear evokes intense and frequent responses from significant others. Thus the more fear and avoidance behavior that a child evokes, the more attention he will receive from significant others. Since fear and avoidance rather than coping responses are consistently rewarded by significant others, the child fails to develop adaptive responses to aversive stimuli. This lack increases his potential to feel afraid and to try to manipulate others to help him avoid the noxious situation. This theory helps to account for the frequent observation of the tyrannical, manipulative, and narcissistic behavior of phobic children (Greenacre, 1952; Hersov, 1960a, 1960b; Leventhal & Sills, 1964) and the problems of distinguishing between "brat" behavior and phobia (Williams, 1959).

Two Factor theory recognizes the validity of both Respondent and Operant social learning explanations and increases the sophistication of the theory. Mowrer (1956) was the first to recognize the need for a combined theory and speculated that phobias originated according to the Respondent conditioning paradigm. Anxiety reduction associated with the noxious stimulus became a secondary reinforcer. Since anxiety is most unpleasant, any behavior that reduces anxiety, such as avoidance of the noxious stimulus, is rewarding. Thus anxiety reduction associated with elimination of the noxious stimulus becomes the operant reward for avoiding the noxious stimulus created by associative conditioning. This theory assumes that phobias are mediated through the autonomic nervous system. However, Soloman et al. (1962) have shown experimentally that behavior is in large part regulated by the central nervous system. Based on Soloman's work and a series of their own studies, Bandura et al. (1969) have advanced a dual process theory which recognizes that threatening stimuli evoke emotional arousal which has both autonomic and central nervous system components, but that the *arousal process* operates primarily at the central level, exercising some degree of control over instrumental avoidance. It follows that if the arousal capacity of subjective threatening events is extinguished, then both the motivation and one set of controlling stimuli for avoidance behavior are removed. This theory has led to a series of studies aimed at eliminating fear behavior which are based on the assumptions that extinction of fear arousal will reduce phobic behavior, that fear arousal can be eliminated on a vicarious level (Modeling), and that the absence of anticipated negative consequences is a requisite condition for fear extinction.

Cognitive development theory is concerned primarily with the interaction between the developing organism and the increasing complexity of his world. While there is no developmental theory of phobia, as such, we have previously noted that certain phobias are more prevalent at specific ages than at others and, that phobias in children tend to disappear more rapidly than in adults. When we discuss treatment we also note that a crucial ingredient in overcoming a phobia is the patient's willingness to confront the stimulus. Developmental theory postulates that maturation affects the way a person perceives and reacts to his environment. We have seen that fear of snakes is absent below the age of two, apparently because the infant has not developed a concept of a snake. We can postulate that the central nervous system has to be sufficiently mature before the person is capable of developing a phobia. Furthermore, the transient quality of phobias in childhood probably reflects a different condition of the organism rather than a difference in the conditioning history or the maintenance reinforcements. Surwillo (1971), has found, for example, that somewhere around the age of 12, the alpha rhythm of the central nervous system matures to an adult level. This phenomena coincides with the age at which school phobias become a more serious problem. It may be that child phobias are actually quite different phenomena from adult phobias, even though there is behavioral similarity.

Developmental theory addresses a point that learning theories tend to minimize: the differential effect of stimuli on subjects. Social learning theories explain an individual's stimulus perceptions on the basis of his unique conditioning history, but clinical evidence suggests that conditioning does not occur on the basis of a simple stimulus-response model. Very seldom does a clinician obtain a history of a uniquely painful situation associated with the onset of the phobia. More typically, the child reports events at onset which have no deleterious effects on many other children who are equally exposed. But the phobic child sees as dangerous a stimulus that most children disregard even though there may be some potential unpleasantness or a low probability of danger (e.g., wind noise and thunderstorms). Such an interpretation of the stimulus does not seem to occur in laboratory conditions, which as a rule take a universally noxious stimulus as the unconditioned one.

The role of the subject's interpretation of the feared stimulus has had little attention in the etiology of phobias. We will not undertake a discussion of the evolution of meaning. However, we suggest that some examples from Piaget may have analogs in the development of childhood phobias.

Piaget (1970) has demonstrated that a child's sense perceptions are based on constructions arising from interaction of subject and object. An example is the construction which enables a nine- to 12-month-old child to discover the permanence of objects. Initially, the child relies on the position of the object in his perceptual field and later permanence occurs independent of any actual perception. During the early months, there are no permanent objects, only perceptual pictures that appear, dissolve, and sometimes reappear. The "permanence" of an object to a child is first demonstrated when the child searches for the object after it has disappeared.

Thus a child is not a passive receiver who ingests the adult's view of the world. Input undergoes significant transformation, the nature of which depends on the child's age. Another example of the child's age-related conception of reality involves the perception of the conservation of quantity of matter across changes in shape. A five-year-old, who has witnessed milk being poured from a short, broad glass into a tall, narrow glass will state that the quantity of milk has increased ("the milk is higher in this glass"). An eight-year-old, though, will state promptly that the amount of milk has not changed across pourings. The eight-year-old's conception of reality includes the notion that quantity is conserved across transformations; the five-year-old's world view does not include this concept.

Thus according to developmental theory objects as perceived by children are age- and state-dependent, as the child's constructions and schema about the nature of reality evolve. Although we have no empirical evidence, we would postulate that a precondition for phobia is a construction of the object as dangerous, and that phobias that occur frequently at certain ages reflect the structuring process typical for that stage in development. Far from being pathognomonic, such fears would be considered a necessary and desirable aspect of development. This line of reasoning suggests that a precondition for treatment is for the patient to wish to be rid of the phobia and to consider the treatment appropriate to his schema of his personal world.

Transactional approaches incorporate elements of the psychoanalytic, developmental, and social learning theories, and, to date, represent no integrated theory. The primary thesis is that social intercourse is critical in the generation and maintenance of pathognomonic behavior. Individuals consciously and unconsciously construct social contracts with one another which form the matrix within which business is "transacted." The social contracts that are set up and the methods used to transact interpersonal business are a function of the individual's present experiencing, his past experience, and his hopes and expectations for the future. These experiences are processed in terms of three cognitive constructs: the individual as child, as parent, and as adult. Thus personality, interpersonal relationships, and psychopathology are viewed as an interaction among these constructs, the social contracts and the methods for transacting business.

The primary contribution of this theory to understanding phobia lies in the importance accorded the mutually influencing relationships of a phobic child and the significant persons in his environment, particularly the mother. We have already noted the explanation advanced by operant theory which emphasizes the reward function of social reinforcers. Transactional approaches incorporate operant principles, assuming that the anticipatory anxiety of parents, the phobic response of the child, and the protective or punishing response of parents are all mutually reinforcing. But it is further postulated that to change the contingencies, some member of the relationship has to decide to renegotiate the social contract and develop other transactional methods. To do this, an internal adjustment within all subsystems would have to occur. Transactionalists postulate that persons involved in a phobia believe that the phobic contract "makes sense" and resist attempts to change it. It makes sense to them not only in terms of the immediate transactions, but also in terms of the balance among their child, adult, and parent subsystems. Thus when parents of a school phobic are asked how they decide to permit a child to stay out of school in defiance of the law, they will explain that the child is "sick" and they do not wish to precipitate a "nervous breakdown." This makes sense to all parties and is the basis of their social contract with one another. The directive from a therapist to return the child to school will usually be resisted unless a new contract can be negotiated that "makes sense." According to this theory, a therapist's job is not one of simply reconditioning a child to a noxious situation, but also entails the renegotiation of a social contract between parent and child (and school).

TREATMENT

In spite of the lack of a generally accepted definition and theory of phobia, a plethora of remedial techniques have been developed in recent years. Advocates of most of these techniques, however, have based their claims upon single cases or uncontrolled studies. Hersen (1971) reviewed the literature on school phobia in 1971 and found that the new behavioral therapies held promise, but he noted the dearth of well-controlled studies upon which to base generalizations. With a few exceptions the same state of affairs is true at this writing. Thus once again we are forced to use the conventional wisdom of clinical experience.

Techniques developed over the past 75 years include interpretation, clarification, catharsis, abreaction, transactional analysis, reciprocal inhibition, hierarchy construction, systematic desensitization, implosion, positive and negative reinforcement, functional analysis, and contingency management. While each of these techniques involves different processes and each has been associated with the alleviation of phobias, the treatment process can be reduced to four basic essentials; establishment of a relationship, clarification of the stimulus, desensitization to the stimulus, and confrontation of the stimulus. This section on the treatment of phobias is organized around these basic processes.

Establishment of a Relationship

Strupp (1973) has stated that one basic condition for therapeutic change is that the "therapist creates and maintains a helping relationship (patterned in significant respects after the parent–child relationship) characterized by respect, interest, understanding, tact, maturity, and a firm belief in his ability to help [p. 1]." Precisely how the therapist creates this relationship, varies with the therapist but most experts believe that a relationship begins and is maintained through interviews with parents and child. Some professionals prefer to interview parents and children separately while others prefer a family group interview. These decisions, however, appear to be more stylistic than crucial in forming a helping relationship.

The initial interview should establish as clearly as possible the history of the phobia, precipitating conditions, previous efforts made by child and parents to reduce the phobia, stimuli controlling the phobia, events within the family that might be related to the phobia (e.g., deaths, changes in locations of home, or a serious illness), and practical questions such as family and community resources, sleeping arrangements, and neighborhood conditions. If the phobia occurs outside the home, the therapist needs to know the context in which the noxious stimulus evokes fear. In the case of a school phobia, for example, one needs to know what has previously been done at school to help the child, the nature of the relationship of parents with school personnel, and what school resources may be available when the child reenters. Some of this information will have to be gathered from the school, but some information can be obtained from the child and parent. During the interview, the therapist also tries to determine which parent is most involved with the child as well as who is most capable of helping the child through the difficult confrontation stage. Also, an assessment of the family transactions at this stage helps the therapist to know how parents reinforce the child's avoidance and dependence behaviors, and what might be done to encourage another type of transactional system.

This information gathering is not only important for treatment planning, but it is a necessary aspect of Strupp's definition of a helping relationship. Being able to relate their problems and express their anxieties and frustrations to an empathetic listener seems to reduce much parental anxiety. By the time parents reach a therapist, they have tried many techniques to help their child and have received much outside help and advice from well-meaning friends and relatives which has not helped but has often created even greater guilt and frustration. Feeling trust and confidence in a therapist goes a long way toward restoring parents' confidence in themselves and in their child. This sense of trust is often further facilitated if parents can voice their own guilt and anxiety arising from the contribution they believe they have made to the child's problems. Often the guilt stems from their own problems which they try not to pass on to their children. This guilt gives rise to compensatory child rearing practices by which the parents attempt to make up to the child unfulfilled needs from their own childhood. As these concerns are voiced and clarified, parents not only separate the present from the past, but also gain greater confidence in the therapist's capacity to help. It is within the context of a helping relationship that the three remaining treatment processes take place.

Stimulus Clarification

The first step in treatment planning is to determine what are the stimuli controlling the phobic behavior. We have already noted from the cases of Sperling (1961) and Smith and Sharpe (1970) that theoretical orientation affects what the therapist selects as discriminative stimuli. At this stage of our knowledge, we believe that an open-minded and pragmatic investigation of the total problem should be carried out before a choice of treatment is decided upon. In addition to the Sperling case in which a connection was made between the mother's operation and school refusal, and Smith and Sharpe's case where fear of class recitation precipitated school refusal, Pittman (1970) reports a case of a 13-year-old school-phobic who resisted all attempts to return to school until a plan was worked out to keep the grandmother in the parent's home rather than placing her in a nursing home. Apparently, the phobia was an attempt to maintain a hidden, possessive relationship with the grandmother which was accidentally discovered when a team from the hospital went to the home to forcibly take the child to school. With the grandmother's cooperation there were no further problems. In another example, Messer (1964) reports a case of family therapy where an eight-year-old school-phobic returned to school after complex family relationships were aired in a family group. Following this revelation, parents were asked to return the child to school, which they did with no further problems. In each of these four examples of successfully treated school-phobics, therapists used a wide range of theoretical orientations and interviewing techniques to ascertain the discriminative stimuli. Furthermore, in one of the few controlled studies of the treatment of clinical level phobias in children, we concluded that the basic therapeutic ingredients alleviating phobic behavior had not as yet been isolated.

Our experience cautions us not to become too committed to the set of stimuli reported by the children as the crucial ones. Children's observations are known to be unreliable, and often they say what they believe adults want to hear rather than what they personally experience. Also, words can carry different meanings for children and adults. We found, for example, that when we asked children if they wanted to be free of their fear, they often said no. This surprised us until we realized that the children thought we were asking if they wanted to confront the feared object. Of course, they did not want to confront the noxious stimulus as long as it produced anxiety. Our words simply meant something different to the children than they meant to us.

In view of these considerations, we believe that clinicians should remain open-minded and should bring to bear all theoretical notions and assessment techniques when determining the stimuli controlling a phobia. This belief does not imply that all possible dynamics and contingencies should be investigated before a treatment plan is formulated, but it does assert that therapists should avoid automatically applying a procedure or technique without thought to the individual characteristics of each case. The determination of the discriminative stimuli and the formulation of the treatment plan demands creative talent from the therapist and the use of the full repertoire of theoretical ideas and technological innovations.

Desensitization to the Stimulus

Desensitization occurs in many ways. Dr. Lucy Jessner, a child analyst in Boston, told of a child with a school phobia who went back to school after an initial visit. Upon inquiry, the mother reported that the child agreed to go back to school if she did not have "to see that woman again."

Wolpe (1958) has developed the most elaborate approach, known as systematic desensitization. This method has been so extensively described in the literature that we mention only the main elements. The basic idea is that a person cannot experience pain and pleasure simultaneously, and that pleasure can inhibit a pain response if the pain is not too severe. Since the object is only psychologically painful, the approach to the stimulus can be made through the imagination. Wolpe adapted a method of muscular relaxation to offset the pain associated with the noxious stimulus. After constructing a stimulus hierarchy, graded from least to most painful, and after the subject has learned muscular relaxation, the therapist presents the least threatening stimulus, asking the child to imagine the stimulus while remaining relaxed. This process continues step-by-step until the most painful stimulus can be imagined in a relaxed state. Systematic desensitization (SDT) has been successfully applied to children (Miller et al., 1972a; Tasto, 1969; Ohler & Terwilliger, 1969; Miller, 1972; Lazarus, 1959). However, the Miller and Ohler studies indicate equivocal superiority of SDT over other types of therapy or even a control group, and Lazarus et al. (1965) cites a case that suggests that SDT should only be employed when high levels of manifest anxiety accompany the phobia. This refinement might improve results, but as we stated previously, we found it impossible to separate respondent from operant conditioned phobias. Furthermore, there are problems with the application of SDT, not the least of which is that it is an extremely boring procedure. Automation certainly has a future with SDT! Sometimes it seems like an absurd process, particularly to adolescents, and sometimes the child may go to sleep, shift the hierarchy, or refuse to fantasize or relax muscles. Since there is no overwhelming evidence of the efficiency of SDT, we suggest that it be incorporated in the therapeutic repertoire as one of many possible desensitization techniques.

Since Wolpe (1958) first described his procedures, many investigations have been undertaken to isolate the critical variables in desensitization. However, it is still not clear how stimuli are actually desensitized. For example, the interpretations made by workers of the analytic school seem to serve as a desensitization process, but the exact mechanism is unknown. It may take place, as analytic theory contends, when an associative connection occurs between an unconscious conflict and the phobic symbol, but it is just as likely that the mechanism involves a psychic shock process which combines emotional arousal with flooding of ideational material similar to that employed in implosive techniques. Whatever the mechanism, case studies suggest that "interpretations" within the context of a clinical interview can serve to desensitize a child, but little is known of the specific conditions under which this occurs.

Other procedures have individual case support. Lazarus and Abramovitz (1962) used a doll play technique called emotive imagery to stimulate fantasy rehearsal of assertive behaviors in school. Conn (1941) describes a more elaborate play technique in which dolls are used to act out fearful fantasies. Conn's case was a nine-year-old who was afraid of being kidnapped and through the doll-play became desensitized.

The newest technique, called Implosive Therapy on this side of the Atlantic and Flooding in England, has a theoretical base similar to systematic desensitization, but instead of a gradual introduction to the stimulus, the subject is exposed in imagery and sometimes *in vivo* to the most intense stimulus in a very short period of time. We could find no systematic studies of implosion with children, although Marks reports that when used with adults this technique achieves the best results of all desensitization procedures. We have already mentioned Smith and Sharpe's (1970) study of a successful implosion of a 13-year-old, and Hersen (1968) reports a case of a periodic school-phobic with a compulsion ritual against disease that was successfully imploded. We imploded three adolescent school-phobics with one success, one partial success, and one failure. For reasons other than the outcome of these efforts, we discontinued our program, but these results do not point to implosion as a panacea. Where systematic desensitization is dull, Implosive Therapy is nerve-wracking when it works well. Once, during the implosion of a case, the therapist broke off the procedure and recommended to observing colleagues that the implosion be stopped and the child hospitalized. He was urged to continue, however, and did so with a successful outcome. This case was greatly helped when the father did an about-face, moved in from the periphery of the family, and took a strong, firm stand against the child's tyrannical behavior. The father's action occurred when the child had again left school after returning following the implosion. This case points to the complexity of psychotherapy and the number of variables involved in changing behavior or attitudes.

Another desensitization technique that bears mentioning is an operant procedure. Ayllon, Smith, and Rogers (1970) discuss the case of an eight-year-old school-phobic girl who was successfully treated by contingency management. A behavioral assessment revealed that Valerie slept one hour later than her siblings and then went to a neighbor's who provided a pleasant and compatible reinforcer to remaining out of school. No particularly unpleasant experiences had occurred at school. Treatment first involved bringing Valerie to school the last 1½ hours of the day, accompanied by an attendant who had established a relationship; then prompting and shaping school attendance through use of primary and secondary reinforcers; and finally withdrawing positive reinforcers and using aversive consequences when not attending. Valerie was back in school in 45 days. Lazarus, Davison, and Polefka (1965) also used a combination of token reinforcement and emotive imagery after an unsuccessful treatment of a nine-year-old with systematic desensitization, and Patterson (1965) reports a successful treatment of school phobia by operant methods. Once again, single case studies make generalizations difficult. One wonders why the elaborate procedures of Ayllon et al. (1970) were necessary in face of the 96% cure rate using clinical methods for this age child. Yet, since the mother was working and there was little adult pressure, an operant technique may have been the therapy of choice. Again, it is a procedure to keep in mind, but it appears very inefficient with young phobics.

A final desensitization method is the use of drugs. Gittelman-Klein and Klein (1971) reported a double blind study of the effects of imipramine (Tofranil) on 35 school phobics, ages six to 14. Children, stratified by age and sex, were randomly assigned to imipramine or placebo pills. Evaluation after six weeks of treatment revealed that 47% of the subjects with placebo returned, but 81% with imipramine returned. This difference was not established until after six weeks of treatment, for during the first three weeks, there was no difference between drug and placebo groups. These investigators also found that there were no age effects, and that the drug group reported much less subjective anxiety than the placebo group. This study needs to be replicated, but the evidence suggests that Tofranil is a powerful desensitizer and may be the most effective method for desensitizing adolescent phobics.

It is often necessary in working with children's phobias to disengage the parents from the phobic process, perhaps even to desensitize them. Almost all writers have noted the close involvement of at least one parent in the child's problem. Very little therapy with parents has been reported although an operant theory of phobia would suggest that the involved parent would be the most advantageous person with whom to work. Also, several studies (Abe, 1972; Hagman, 1932; Hersov, 1960a) have found that many parents have phobias which could serve as models for their children. Bandura's (1967) work on modeling and vicarious learning lends credence to the idea that phobic children may be imitating phobic parents.

We had one case of an eight-year-old girl who periodically refused to go to school, manifesting the usual signs of terror that baffled the mother and school personnel. This was the only child of an older couple. The mother had worked for years, but was delighted at the birth of her daughter, not only because she had always wanted children, which many miscarriages had prevented, but also because she had always wanted to give to her child many of the things that she had missed in growing up. The mother felt close to her parents, but also exploited by them because of the illness of her mother and the selfishness of her father and brothers. Even as an adult, she was the only child who took care of her parents, but still she felt they favored her brothers. Despite the family conflict, her only real problems occurred in adolescence when she felt unappreciated by her teachers despite the fact that she worked hard at her studies. Several instances in which teachers had embarrassed her were recalled with a vividness as if they had occurred yesterday. She was determined that her daughter was not going to have to repeat her experiences. To avoid this, she made sure that her daughter had all the material advantages and was never exploited at home, although she did not spoil her in the usual sense of the word. The daughter was the center of parental interest and affection, and every slight by peers or teachers was deeply felt by mother. Mother also went to school with some regularity to ensure that her daughter was not abused as she felt she had been.

In the course of 12 hours of therapy, this mother painfully reexperienced those events of her past and connected them to her current inability to let her daughter work out her own relationships with her peers and teachers. Behind it all was a conflict between the ideal mother of her dreams and the woman and mother she now realized she must be to help her child. The dream mother which she had tried to be was the all-giving, self-sacrificing, fiercely protecting mother; the opposite of her own self-pitying, sickly, and exploitive mother. The reality mother had been an efficient and highly respected career woman, who, now as a housewife, was resentful when her husband and child went into the exciting world. Moreover, she was afraid to stay alone in the house. She usually finished her work by 10:00 A.M. and then had nothing to do with her energy and talents except to worry about her daughter and mull over the past rejections. As she faced this conflict and released the past, she decided to go back to work and let her daughter fight her own battles. Almost like magic, when mother decided she no longer needed the daughter, the daughter decided she no longer needed mother. It was, however, with the ambivalence of pride and fear that she related in the last therapeutic session, with a smile and a tear, the sight of her only child going out on Hallowe'en night with her friends "tricking and treating."

This case, of course, argues for the thesis that separation anxiety is the basis of school phobia, but the point here is that the child's fear of school was diminished partially by desensitizing mother to the hurts of her own past. It was the child's resistance to school that was the stimulus for mother to recall her own past and face the major conflict in her current life. However, as the mother did this, she was able to help her daughter master the anxiety associated with school and her relationships with her peers. Even though the child was never seen in therapy, the mother was helping the child to confront and desensitize the school as a noxious stimulus.

In brief, there appear to be a number of techniques available to help a child desensitize noxious stimuli, including systematic desensitization, implosion, emotive imagery, doll-play, interpretation, operant conditioning, family therapy, tranquilizing drugs, and parent therapy. Each of these methods must be applied within the context of a relationship, and each must be associated with a continuous and eventually successful confrontation of the stimulus by the child.

Confrontation of the Stimulus

The last essential element in the treatment of phobia is stimulus confrontation. All research and clinical experience suggests that confrontation is an absolutely necessary aspect of treatment, as well as a measure of its success. In the presence of the stimulus, the child learns how not to be afraid or learns that he is no longer anxious. All investigators believe that phobias will not dissipate through time alone, but rather by a process of direct confrontation with the noxious stimulus. Differences arise only as to when and how the confrontation should take place.

Central to confrontation is attitude. In our experience, parents are usually ambivalent about a confrontation. Consciously, they recognize that the child needs to sleep in his own bed, to go to school, or to be comfortable during a thunderstorm, but they will also have many reasons why the child should not be forced to confront any of these stimuli. In our experience, there comes a point in all successful treatment when at least one parent resolves this ambivalence and decides that no matter what comes, the child will confront the stimuli and that they will not feel sorry or guilty at having forced the confrontation. This resolution of ambivalence is true for parents of both young and older children and is a critical ingredient in arranging a confrontation. We seldom see such dramatic attitude changes in children. Generally, children are initially opposed to all confrontation and only gradually and incidentally do they mention that they now do with ease what a few weeks previously had been done with such anguish.

It is generally unwise to expect a child to confront voluntarily a noxious experience early in treatment, because they do not recognize the long-range advantages. As desensitization proceeds and as parents become less and less involved, we find that with skill and planning, the children will make the effort to confront. Therapists need to realize that not all efforts succeed immediately and in cases where continuous confrontation is not possible, further desensitization will be necessary. It is a creative act on the part of the therapist to judge when a child and his parents are ready for confrontation and to employ the necessary supports to help at the critical time. In the case of school phobia, advance planning with school personnel is usually helpful. We like to secure the service of someone at school that will receive the child when the parents arrive so that separation is swift and sure. This person can also help the child into the classroom. Occasionally, a room near the principal's office can be provided for the child if the panic in the classroom gets too severe. Our experience, however, suggests that all of these auxilliary supports should be used sparingly, since the main message is that the schoolroom is a safe place and that the child is expected to stay and do his work just like everyone else. We seek to provide the school personnel with professional support through the initial crisis and to guide them so that they treat the child matter-of-factly, remain calm in face of the child's fear, temper, or tears, and give the child time to master his anxiety without becoming the focus of either special privileges or animosity. Once parent and school personnel realize that confrontation is necessary and will not provoke disastrous effects and that a caring but calm attitude helps the child gain control, then the phobic reaction usually dissipates. If it does not, then the therapist has to weigh the possible advantage of continuing the confrontation against the ability of others to tolerate the phobic reaction. In case of older phobics one often has to resort to hospitalization or to tranquilizing drugs. As mentioned earlier, hospitalization is reported in the literature as being a successful method of confronting parents and children with their separation anxiety, but in our experience, we have seen no better results with hospitalization than with out-patient treatment. We want to stress, however, that there is little research upon which to base these judgments.

Kennedy (1965) prefers a management approach with Type I school-phobics in which the therapist maximizes influence variables by leading the interview, being optimistic, emphasizing success, and presenting a formula. This formula includes a moratorium on all topics related to school, a deemphasis on somatic complaints, a forced reentry of the child on the following Monday morning with the least involved parent taking the child to school, matter of fact approval, compliments to the child on the first night for attending school, and a party on Wednesday for successful attendance.

Kennedy seems to be saying that if the parent's confidence can be restored by these simple techniques then the therapist does not have to deal with all the other complicated issues. On the other hand, other techniques such as Sperling's interpretation or Jessner's single interview resulted in the child returning to school without Kennedy's management techniques. Thus many methods seem to work, and we again urge a selection of the method to fit the case.

Some professionals advocate the use of the juvenile court as a means for forcing confrontation. Our experience argues against this procedure for many reasons, but basically it is cumbersome, has many undesirable side consequences, and we know of no instances when it has been effective. Even the threat is of no value because phobics do not anticipate logical consequences. Therefore, we urge this solution to be dropped, as well as all threats because they seem to increase anxiety and withdrawal behavior. Even hospitalization should not be used as a threat, but rather presented when all other alternatives have been exhausted. In brief, we find that threats and punishment are ineffective methods in helping a child to become desensitized to a noxious stimulus. If desensitization cannot be accomplished by means discussed in this chapter, than resorting to punishment represents the final failure and becomes an outlet for therapist resentment and frustration.

Orchestrating a confrontation requires the full range of therapeutic imagination and creativity. We have already seen how Sperling used interpretation and suggestion to get the child to go back to school, while in Messner's case the suggestion was made in the context of a discussion of family dynamics. In the Allyon et al. case an elaborate reward system was worked out, combined with aversive stimuli, while Smith and Sharpe imploded their child with verbal imagery until he was willing to confront the stimuli *in vivo*.

In our own study we used virtually every conceivable procedure to prepare the child for a confrontation with the feared stimulus. A partial list of procedures would include systematic desensitization, interpretations, and ensuring that the consequences of avoidance were as noxious as possible (e.g., removing television and insisting the child stay in bed if he were not in school). We found that all of these procedures worked, and all of them failed to work. Hence we would respond with skepticism to any statement linking a specific technique to a successful outcome. A clinician has to discover, often by trial and error, the appropriate technique for the specific case.

In brief, confrontation is a necessary step in the treatment of phobia. It can be done only when parents have resolved their ambivalence, and when other persons in the situation can receive the child without getting involved in the child's manipulative and phobic reactions. The therapist must continuously judge whether child, parent, and environment are ready for the confrontation and once it is begun, every effort should be made to bring it to a successful conclusion lest the child's avoidance be reestablished.

REFERENCES

Abe, K. Phobias and nervous symptoms in childhood and maturity: Persistence and associations. *British Journal of Psychiatry,* 1972, **120,** 275–283.

Adams, P. L. Bisexual conflicts of adolescents with school phobia. *Psychiatry Digest,* 1970, 48–49.

Achenbach, T. M. The classification of children's psychiatric symptoms: A factor analytic study. *Psychological Monograph,* 1966, **80** (6) (Whole Nq. 615).

Agras, W. Stewart, Chapin, H. N., & Oliveau, D. C. The natural history of phobia. *Archives of General Psychiatry,* 1972, **26,** 315–317.

Arieti, S. A re-examination of the phobic symptom and of symbolism in psychopathology. *American Journal of Psychiatry,* 1961, **118,** 106–110.

Ayllon, T., Smith, D., & Rogers, M. Behavioral management of school phobia. *Journal of Behavioral Therapy and Experimental Psychiatry,* 1970, **1,** 125–138.

Bandura, A., Blanchard, E. B., & Ritter,B. Relative efficacy of desensitization and modeling approaches for inducing behavioral, affective, and attitudinal changes. *Journal of Desensitization and Modeling,* 1969, **13,** 173–199.

Bandura, A., Grusec, J. E., & Menlove, F. L. *Vicarious extinction of avoidance behavior. Journal of Personality and Social Psychology,* 1967, **5,** 16–23.

Barker, P. The in-patient treatment of school refusal. *British Journal of Medical Psychology,* 1968, **41,** 381.

Berecz, J.M. Phobias of childhood: Etiology and treatment. *Psychological Bulletin,* 1968, **70,** 694–720.

Berg, I. A follow-up study of school phobic adolescents admitted to an in-patient unit. *Journal of Child Psychology and Psychiatry,* 1970, **2,** 37–47.

Berg, I., & McGuire, R. Are school phobic adolescents overdependent? *British Journal of Psychiatry,* 1971, **119,** 167–168.

Berg, I., Nichols, K., & Pritchard, C. School phobia—Its classification and relationship to dependency. *Journal of Child Psychology and Psychiatry,* 1969, **10,** 123–141.

Bolman, W. M. Systems theory, psychiatry, and school phobia. *American Journal of Psychiatry,* 1970, **127,** 25–32.

Bowlby, J. Separation anxiety: A critical review of the literature. *Journal of Child Psychology and Psychiatry,* 1960, **1,** 251–269.

Bornstein, B. Phobia in a two-and-a-half year old child. *Psychoanalytic Quarterly,* 1935, **4,** 93–119.

Caldwell, B. M., & Honig, A. Approach: A procedure for patterning responses of adults and children, JSAS. *Catalog of Selected Documents in Psychology*, 1971, **1** (Ms. 2).

Castaneda, A., McCandless, B. R., & Palermo, D. S. The children's form of the manifest anxiety scale. *Child Development*, 1956, **16**, 317–326.

Cattell, R., & Coan, R. W. Personality factors in middle childhood as revealed in parent ratings. *Child Development*, 1957, **28**, 439–458.

Colm, H. N. Phobias in Children. *Psychoanalysis and the Psychoanalytic Review*, 1959, **46**, 65–84.

Conn, J. H. The treatment of fearful children. *The American Journal of Orthopsychiatry*, 1941, **2**, 744–751.

Coolidge, J. C., Brodie, R. D., & Feeney, B. A 10-year follow-up study of 66 school phobic children. *American Journal of Orthopsychiatry*, 1964, **34**, 675–695.

Coolidge, J. C., Hahn, P. B., & Peck, A. L. School phobia: Neurotic crisis or way of life. *American Journal of Orthopsychiatry*, 1957, **27**, 296–306.

Coolidge, J. C., Tessman, E., Waldfogel, S., & Willer, M. L. School phobia in adolescence: A manifestation of severe character disturbance. *American Journal of Orthopsychiatry*, 1960, **30**, 483–494.

Dixon, J. J., deMonchaux, C., & Sandler, J. Patterns of anxiety: The phobias. *British Journal of Medical Psychology*, 1957, **30**, 34–40.

Dreger, R. M., Lewis, P. M., Rich, T. A., & Miller, K. S. Behavior classification project. *Journal of Consulting Psychology*, 1964, **28**, 1–13.

Eisenberg, L. School phobia: A study in the communication of anxiety. *American Journal of Psychiatry*, 1958, **114**, 712. (a)

Eisenberg, L., School phobia: Diagnosis, genesis and clinical management. *Pediatric Clinics of North America*, 1958, **5**, 645–666. (b)

Errera, P., & Coleman, J. V. A long-term follow-up study of neurotic phobic patients in a psychiatric clinic. *Journal of Nervous and Mental Disease*, 1963, **136**, 267.

Fogarty, J. P. School phobia—A preliminary report on 57 cases. *Journal of the Irish Medical Association*, 1971, **64**, 72–75.

Franks, C. M., & Susskind, D. J. Behavior modification with children: Rationale and technique. *Journal of School Psychology*, 1968, **4**, 75–86.

Freud, S., Analysis of a phobia in a five-year-old boy. *Complete Psychological Works*, Vol. 10. London: Hogarth Press, 1962. Pp. 101–147.

Gelder, M. G., & Marks, I. M. Different ages of onset in varieties of phobia. *American Journal of Psychiatry*, 1966, **123**, 128.

Gittelman-Klein, R., & Klein, D. Controlled imipramine treatment of school phobia. *Archives of General Psychiatry*, 1971, **25**, 204–207.

Glick, B. S. Conditioning therapy with phobic patients: Success and failure. *American Journal of Psychotherapy*, 1970, **24**, 92–101.

Greenacre, P. *Trauma, growth and personality*. New York: W. W. Norton, 1952.

Hagman, E. R. A study of fears of children of pre-school age. *Journal of Experimental Education*, 1932, **1**, 110–130.

Hampe, E., Noble, H., Miller, L. C., & Barrett, C. L. Phobic children one and two years posttreatment. *Journal of Abnormal Psychology*, 1973, **82**, 446–453.

Hellman, I. Hampstead nursery follow-up studies: Sudden separation and its effect followed over twenty years. *Psychoanalytic Study of the Child*, 1962, **17**, 159–174.

Hersen, M. Treatment of a compulsive and phobic disorder through a total behavior therapy program: A case study. *Psychotherapy: Theory, Research and Practice*, 1968, **5**, 220–224.

Hersen, M. Behavior modification approach to a school phobia case. *Journal of Clinical Psychology*, 1970, **26**, 128–132.

Hersen, M. The behavioral treatment of school phobia. *The Journal of Nervous and Mental Disease*, 1971, **153**, 2.

Hersov, L. A. Persistent non-attendance at school. *Journal of Child Psychology and Psychiatry*, 1960, **1**, 130–136. (a)

Hersov, L. A. Refusal to go to school. *Journal of Child Psychology and Psychiatry*, 1960, **1**, 137–145. (b)

Irwin, O. C., The latent time of body startle in infants. *Child Development*, 1932, **3**, 104–107.

Ivey, E. P. Recent advances in the psychiatric diagnosis and treatment of phobias. *American Journal of Psychiatry*, 1959, **13**, 35–50.

Jarvis, V. Countertransference in the management of school phobia. *Psychoanalytic Quarterly*, 1964, **33**, 411–419.

Jersild, A. T., & Holmes, F. B. Children's fears. *Child development*, 1935, Monograph 20.

Johnson, A. M., Falstein, E. I., Szurek, S. A., & Svendsen, M. School phobia. *American Journal of Orthopsychiatry*, 1941, **11**, 702–711.

Jones, H. E., & Jones, M. C. A study of fear. *Childhood Education*, 1928, **5**, 136–143.

Kennedy, W. A. School phobia: Rapid treatment of fifty cases. *Journal of Abnormal Psychology*, 1965, **70**, 285–289.

Klein, D. F., & Klein, R. G. School phobia: Diagnostic considerations in the light of imipramine effects, unpublished paper.

Klein, E. The reluctance to go to school. *The Psychoanalytic Study of the Child*, 1945, **1**, 263–281.

L'Abate, L. Personality correlates of manifest anxiety in children. *Journal of Consulting Psychology*, 1960, **24**, 342–348.

Lader, M. H. Palmar skin conductance measures in anxiety and phobic states. *Journal of Psychosomatic Research*, 1967, **2**, 271–281.

Lacey, J. I. Psychophysiological approaches to the evaluation of psychotherapeutic process and outcome. In F. Rubenstein & M. B. Perloff (Eds.), *Research in psychology*. Washington, D.C.: American Psychological Association, 1958.

Lang, P. J. Fear reduction and fear behavior, patterns in treating a construct. Presented in 3rd Conference in Research in Psychotherapy, Chicago, Ill., June 1966.

Lang, P. J., & Lasovik, A. D. Experimental desensitization of a phobia. *Journal of Abnormal and Social Psychology*, 1963, **66**, 519–525.

Lang, P. J., Melamed, B. G., & Hart, J. A psychophysiological analysis of fear modification using an automated desensitization procedure. *Journal of Abnormal Psychology*, 1970, **76**, 220–234.

Lapousse, R., & Monk, M. A. Fears and worries in a representative sample of children. *American Journal of Orthopsychiatry*, 1959, **29**, 223–248.

Lazarus, A. A. The elimination of children's phobias by deconditioning. In H. J. Eysenck (Ed.), *Behavior therapy and the neuroses*. Oxford: Pergamon Press, 1959.

Lazarus, A. A., & Abramovitz, A. The use of "emotive imagery" in the treatment of children's phobias. *Journal of Mental Science*, 1962, **108**, 191–195.

Lazarus, A. A., Davison, G. C., & Polefka, D. A. Classical and operant factors in the treatment of school phobia. *Journal of Abnormal Psychology*, 1965, **70**, 225–229.

Leitenberg, H., Agras, S., Butz, R., & Wincze, J. Relationship between heart rate and behavioral change during the treatment of phobias. *Journal of Abnormal Psychology*, **1971**, 59–68.

Leton, D. A. Assessment of school phobia. *Mental Hygiene*, 1962, **46**, 256–264.

Leventhal, T., & Sills, M. Self-image in school phobia. *American Journal of Orthopsychiatry*, 1964, **34**, 685–695.

Leventhal, T., Weinberger, G., Stander, R. J., & Stearns, R. P. Therapeutic strategies with school phobics. *American Journal of Orthopsychiatry*, 1967, **37**, 64–70.

Levitt, E. E. *The psychology of anxiety*. Indianapolis: Bobbs-Merrill 1967.

MacFarlane, J. W., Allen, L., & Honzik, M. P. A developmental study of the behavior problems of normal children between twenty-one months and fourteen years. In *University of California Publications in Child Development*. Vol. 2. Berkeley: University of California Press, 1954.

Marks, I. M. *Fears and phobias*. New York: American Press, 1969.

Marks, I. M. The classification of phobic disorders. *British Journal of Psychiatry*, 1970, **116**, 377–386.

Marks, I. M. Phobic disorders four years after treatment: A prospective follow-up. *British Journal of Psychiatry*, 1971, **118**, 683–688.

McCandless, B. R., & Castaneda, A. Anxiety in children, school achievement, and intelligence. *Child Development*, 1956, **27**, 379–382.

Messer, A. A. Family treatment of a school phobic child. *Archives General Psychology*, 1964, **2**, 548.

Miller, D. L. School phobia: Diagnosis, emotional genesis, and management. *New York State Journal of Medicine*, 1972, **72**, 1160–1165.

Miller, L. C. Louisville Behavior Check List for males 6–12 years of age. *Psychological Reports*, 1967, **21**, 885–896.

Miller, L. C. School behavior Check List: An inventory of deviant behavior for elementary school children. *Journal of Consulting and Clinical Psychology*, 1972, **38**, 134–144.

Miller, L. C., Hampe, E., Barrett, C. L., & Noble, H. Children's deviant behavior within the general population. *Journal of Consulting and Clinical Psychology*, 1971 **34**, 16–22. (a)

Miller, L. C., Barrett, C. L., Hampe, E., & Noble, H. Revised anxiety scales for the Louisville Behavior Check List. *Psychology Reports*, 1971, **29**, 503–511. (b)

Miller, L. C., Barrett, C. L., Hampe, E., & Noble, H. Comparison of reciprocal inhibition, psychotherapy, and waiting list control for phobic children. *Journal of Abnormal Psychology*, 1972, **79**, 269–279. (a)

Miller, L. C., Barrett, C. L., Hampe, E., & Noble, H. Factor structure of childhood fears. *Journal of Consulting and Clinical Psychology*, 1972, **39**, 264–268. (b)

Miller, P. M. The use of visual imagery and muscle relaxation in the counterconditioning of a phobic child: A case study. *The Journal of Nervous and Mental Disease*, 1972, **154**, 457–460.

Mowrer, O. H. Two-factor learning theory reconsidered, with special reference to secondary reinforcement and the concept of habit. *Psychological Review*, 1956, **63**, 114–128.

Nichols, K. A., & Berg, I. School phobia and self-evaluation. *Journal of Child Psychology and Psychiatry*, 1970, **2**, 133–141.

Obler, M., & Terwilliger, R. F. Pilot study on the effectiveness of systematic desensitization among children with phobic disorders. *Proceedings, 1969, APA Presentation.*

Patterson, G. R. A learning theory approach to the treatment of the school phobic child. In L. P. Ullmann & L. Krasner (Eds.), *Case studies in behavior modification.* New York: Holt, Rinehart, & Winston, 1965.

Patterson, G. R., Ray, R. S., & Shaw, D. A. Direct intervention in families of deviant children. *Oregon Research Institute Research Bulletin*, 1968, **8**, (9).

Peterson, D. R. Behavior problems of middle childhood. *Journal of Consulting Psychology*, 1961, **25**, 205–209.

Piaget, J. Piaget's theory. In P. H. Mussen (Ed.), *Manual of child psychology.* (3rd ed.) New York: Wiley, 1970. Pp. 703–732.

Pittman, F. S., III. Critical incident No. 7. *International Psychiatric Clinic*, 1970, **7**, 335–341.

Rachman, A., & Costello, C. G. The aetiology and treatment of children's phobias: A review. *American Journal of Psychiatry*, 1961, **118**, 97–105.

Renik, O. Cognitive ego function in the phobic symptom. *Psychoanalytic Quarterly*, 1972, **41**, 537–555.

Rodriguez, A., Rodriguez, M., & Eisenberg, L. The outcome of school phobia: A follow-up study based on 41 cases. *American Journal of Psychiatry*, 1959, **116**, 540–544.

Sarason, S. B., Davidson, K. S., Lighthall, F. F., Waite, R. R., & Ruebush, B. K. *Anxiety in elementary school children.* New York: Wiley 1960.

Sarason, S. B., & Gordon, E. M. The test anxiety questionnaire: Scoring norms. *Journal of Abnormal & Social Psychology*, 1953, **48**, 447–448.

Scherer, M. W., & Nakamura, C. Y. A fear survey schedule for children (FSS-FC): A factor analytic comparison with manifest anxiety (CMAS). *Behavior Research and Therapy*, 1968, **6**, 173–182.

Schmitt, B. D. Diagnosis and treatment: School phobia—the great imitator: A pediatrician's viewpoint. *Pediatrics*, 1971, **48**, 443–451.

Shirley, M. M. *The first two years*. Vol. 2. Minneapolis: University of Minnesota Press, 1933.

Smith, R. E., & Sharpe, T. M. Treatment of a school phobia with implosive therapy. *Journal of Consulting and Clinical Psychology*, 1970, **35**, 239–243.

Smith, S. L. School refusal with anxiety: A review of sixty-three cases. *Canadian Psychiatric Association Journal*, 1970, **15**, 257–264.

Soloman, R. L., & Turner, L. H. Discriminative classical conditioning in dogs paralyzed by curare can later control discriminative avoidance responses in the normal state. *Psychology Review*, 1962, **69**, 202–219.

Sperling, M. Analytic first aid in school phobias. *Psychoanalytic Quarterly*, 1961, **30**, 504–518.

Strupp, H. H. On the basic ingredients of psychotherapy. *Journal of Consulting and Clinical Psychology*, 1973, **41**, 1–8.

Surwillo, W. W. Human reaction time and period of the EGG in relation to development. *Psychophysiology*, 1971, **8**, 468–481.

Tasto, D. Case histories and shorter communications: Systematic desensitization, muscle relaxation and visual imagery in the counterconditioning of four-year-old phobic child. *Behavior Research and Therapy*, 1969, **7**, 409–411.

Terhune, W. B. The phobic syndrome. *Archives of Neurology and Psychiatry*, 1949, **62**, 162–172.

Tucker, W. I. Diagnosis and treatment of the phobic reaction. *American Journal of Psychiatry*, 1956, **112**, 825–830.

Valentine, C. W. The innate bases of fear. *Journal of Genetic Psychology*, 1930, **37**, 394–419.

Waldfogel, S., Coolidge, J. C., & Hahn, P. B. The development, meaning and management of school phobia. *American Journal of Orthopsychiatry*, 1957, **27**, 754–780.

Waldfogel, S., Tessman, E., & Hahn, P. B. Learning problems: A program for early intervention in school phobia. *American Journal of Orthopsychiatry*, 1959, **29**, 342–332.

Walk, R. D. Self ratings of fear in a fear invoking situation. *Journal of Abnormal and Social Psychology*, 1956, **52**, 171–178.

Watson, J., & Rayner, R. Conditioned emotional reactions. *Journal of Experimental Psychology*, 1920, **3**, 1–14.

Waugh, M. Psychoanalytic thought on phobia: Its evolution and its relevance for therapy. *American Journal of Psychiatry*, 1967, **123**, 1075–1080.

Wehr, T. Assessment of children's phobias in a clinic population; Identifying a phobia in a clinical population, (two unpublished manuscripts).

Weiss, M., & Burke, A. A 5 to 10 year follow-up of hospitalized school phobic children and adolescents. *American Journal of Orthopsychiatry,* 1970, **40,** 672–676.

Weiss, M., & Cain, B. The residential treatment of children and adolescents with school phobia. *American Journal of Orthopsychiatry,* 1964, **34,** 103–114.

Williams, C. D. The elimination of tantrum behavior by extinction procedures. *The Journal of Abnormal & Social Psychology,* 1959, **2,** 269.

Wilson, G. D. An electrodermal technique for the study of phobias. *N.Z. Medical Journal,* 1966, **65,** 696–698.

Wolpe, J. *Psychotherapy by reciprocal inhibition.* Stanford, Calif.: Stanford University Press, 1958.

Wolpe, J., & Rachman, S. Psychoanalytic "evidence": A critique based on Freud's case of Little Hans. *Journal of Nervous and Mental Disorders,* 1960, **131,** 135–148.

PART TWO

Childhood Psychoses

CHAPTER 4

Infantile Autism: Status and Research

BERNARD RIMLAND

The scientific and medical literature on the childhood psychoses is confusing and contradictory in numerous respects. There is hardly a topic within the field about which the various authors agree. Some books and articles are written from the psychogenic point of view, as though it were quite well-established that faulty mother–child relations were the sole cause, or at least a major contributing cause, of psychosis in childhood (e.g., Bettelheim, 1967; Ekstein, 1971; Szurek & Berlin, 1973; Tustin, 1972). Other authors concern themselves with biological approaches, and pay scant, if any, attention to the convictions of the psychogenecists (e.g., Boullin, Coleman, & O'Brien, 1970; Himwich, Jenkins, Fujimori, Narasimhacari, & Ebersole, 1972; Ritvo, Yuwiler, Geller, Ornitz, Saeger, & Plotkin, 1970). Actually, the disagreement as to cause of psychosis in children is beginning to be dispelled, since as I noted a decade ago (Rimland, 1964), so much evidence is accumulating against the psychogenic viewpoint that the ranks of the adherents of this viewpoint are thinning rapidly.

Another area of major disagreement relates to the matter of diagnosis. The problem is not so much one of distinguishing the psychotic child from the retarded or the learning-disabled child, although some confusion exists on this point, but instead involves differentiating one type of childhood psychotic from the others. The terms childhood schizophrenia, psychotic child, autistic child, and child with infantile autism have been used so often interchangeably, even by authors who would be expected to know better, that some researchers entering the field with a serious interest in the subject have found the topic so muddled that they have given up in despair. Scientific progress is impeded severely by this chaotic situation. I have devoted a good deal of my attention to an attempt to clarify the diagnostic problem. While I cannot claim to have achieved more than partial success, a good deal has been accomplished, as seen later in this chapter.

The following pages are addressed to several of the more important sources of confusion in the literature on the childhood psychoses. In particular, because of its unusual significance from both the theoretical and practical standpoints, the major focus of attention is upon the small and unique subgroup of psychotic children afflicted with infantile autism.

THE DIAGNOSIS OF INFANTILE AUTISM

Several large-scale intensive surveys in the United States and England have established that the incidence of psychosis in children is about five cases per 10,000 births (Lotter, 1967; Treffert, 1970). The incidence of five children per 10,000 pertains to all forms of psychoses, that is, to the group which is often labelled childhood schizophrenia. The term childhood schizophrenia is not meant to imply a direct relationship to adult schizophrenia, which is different in its manifestations, and very much more common, but only to suggest by analogy that the childhood disorder also produces disorientation and bizarre inappropriate behavior, and is totally or nearly totally disabling.*

In 1943, Leo Kanner, who was then professor of child psychiatry at Johns Hopkins Medical School, published a paper (Kanner, 1943) in which he described in detail 11 psychotic children he had seen over the preceding years. These 11 children were similar in many respects to the children described by many other writers as childhood schizophrenics; Kanner insisted, however, and has continued to insist (e.g., Kanner, 1943, 1958, 1973), that despite the superficial resemblance between those children and the others, there was a remarkable homogeneity of behavior in these 11, and some important differences between them and the previously described children who had been called childhood schizophrenics.

The following year Kanner (1944) described several more children who closely resembled his first group, and this time he named the new category of childhood psychosis—he titled his paper "Early Infantile Autism."

The words early infantile referred to the fact that the disorder was usually present at birth, and was, in his opinion "inborn." The word autistic was used to describe one of the most striking characteristics of the children, their remote, inaccessible personalities, which in some ways made them resemble autistic (daydreaming) adults. The word autism proved to be a poor choice, as Kanner has recently (1973) emphasized, because it led many psychologists and psychiatrists (e.g., Bettelheim, 1967) to conclude, incorrectly, that since autism in

---

*In my book *Infantile Autism*, I referred to nonautistic psychotic children as "childhood schizophrenics," making it clear that the latter term was felt to encompass a number of disorders rather than being a unitary disease. I now prefer to use the term autistic-type children rather than childhood schizophrenics because the latter term implies that we have information that we actually lack. The terms autistic, infantile autism, and classically autistic are used interchangeably.

adults was essentially voluntary, the "autistic" children too were biologically normal individuals who had voluntarily chosen to disassociate themselves from reality, because their dream life was more satisfactory to them than was reality. There is in fact no evidence whatever that infantile autism is voluntary.

When I first met Leo Kanner in 1962 I asked him what proportion of the psychotic children, loosely called autistic by others, were in fact afflicted with infantile autism, as *he* used the term. After a long, thoughtful puff on his ever-present cigar he told me, "Only about 10 percent of the children who have childhood schizophrenia and have therefore been carelessly labelled as "autistic" are really cases of infantile autism." I dutifully recorded his estimate in my book *Infantile Autism* (1964, p. 18). Ten years later, having collected detailed case history material for well over 4000 psychotic children from all over the world, I found Kanner to have been remarkably accurate in his estimate: out of every 100 children showing the bizarre and profound behaviors characteristic of the so-called autistic child, only 10 will, after careful investigation, prove to be bona fide cases of early infantile autism. Thus the incidence of true or classical autism is about five per 100,000, or one birth in 20,000.

Kanner has protested repeatedly against the loose and indiscriminate use of the diagnosis "autistic" and "infantile autism." He has deplored "the dilution of the concept of early infantile autism," and observed that "the diagnosis has been made much too prodigiously." He quite correctly argued:

There is, of course, no denying that overlapping symptomatology creates problems in trying to distinguish between different illnesses which have a number of features in common. But the problem is definitely not solved by the decree that the sharing of symptoms makes the diseases identical or that, because of the partial resemblance, a differentiation is unnecessary [1958, p. 142]."

Both in my book *Infantile Autism,* and in my article (1968) written to commemorate the 25th anniversary of Kanner's first article on autism, I have added my voice to Kanner's, protesting that much of the published literature on the topic was virtually useless because so many authors lumped together heterogeneous subgroups of psychotic children, calling them all autistic. Many authors cite Kanner's classic papers on autism, then blithely proceed to claim that their single case, or all five or all 20 of the children in their sample, were cases of classical autism. Such claims are easily dismissed, in most cases, by careful reading of the case history of the single cases, or, where there are multiple cases, by noting that the authors usually make no mention of the natural control group of nine or so nonautistic psychotic children they had to examine to find each true autistic case.

The concern that Kanner and I have expressed about the loose use of the term autism does not stem from petulance, pedantry, or semantic nitpicking. The history of medicine makes it clear that "nosology precedes etiology." As Kanner has pointed out, little progress could be made toward defeating "the fevers," until the fevers could be separated and treated in terms of the component individual diseases, such as malaria, cholera, diptheria, and tuberculosis.

An example much closer at hand may be found in the remarkable progress made in recent years on the problem of mental retardation. Well over 100 syndromes are now recognizable, and as each has been isolated from the others, it becomes the target for researchers dedicated to finding effective means for remediation or prevention. There is no doubt in my mind but that progress on prevention and remediation of the childhood psychoses has been impeded—I would even go so far as to say halted—by the virtual stalemate that exists in the area of diagnosis. It is certain that there are a *number* of causes of the childhood psychoses, and that the various causes lead to different syndromes. Little progress can be expected until these syndromes can be identified.

In view of the importance of the matter of diagnosis, and the dismal state of diagnostic practice in the area of the childhood psychoses, it is distressing to see the careless and indiscriminate neglect of the one breakthrough that has occurred in this area—Kanner's incisive delineation of infantile autism.

The first part of this chapter is devoted to a brief overview of the syndrome of autism and of Kanner's finding of unusual intelligence in the parents of cases of true autism. Little documentation is provided for these topics, since my book *Infantile Autism* provides the needed references. Following the review a report of recent findings that relate to the areas of controversy is presented.

THE SYNDROME OF AUTISM

At birth the child who later turns out to be a case of classical early infantile autism (Kanner's syndrome) seems to be an unusually healthy and attractive baby. In some instances, the baby seems to be exceedingly alert, almost precociously intelligent in appearance. These hyperalert children tend, by and large, to be those who develop early speech, although their speech is of the peculiarly noncommunicative, autistic variety. Another subgroup of the children who later turn out to be classically autistic tend to be quite passive and inattentive soon after birth.* The parents tend to regard these passive children as particularly "good" babies. This latter subgroup of babies tends to develop into the mute form of autism, in which speech does not occur in early life at all, and in many instances the mute autistic child goes into adolescence and through adulthood without ever uttering a word.

Although Kanner's early papers refer to the fact that some of the children

---

*It is possible that these subgroups among autistic children represent variants in the same sense in which there are at least three types of mongolism and four of PKU.

did develop speech and some did not, the finding that the speaking variety of autism tends to be different in appearance and personality at birth from the non-speaking children is an outgrowth of my own research on my Diagnostic Check List, Form E-2, which is described later.

If the mother has had children before or is used to children, she may notice immediately that the child with autism does not adapt itself to her body and cuddle the way a normal infant does. However, since all babies are different, even experienced parents usually do not become concerned until perhaps the fourth month, which typically finds the normal baby reaching out for its mother when she approaches. The child with autism fails to show any sign of awareness of his mother, or of other people in the environment for that matter. Head-banging is a frequent complaint seen in the case histories of autistic children. Sometimes the child will bang his head against the crib or other objects. Sometimes the head-banging will take place against the body or face of the adult who is holding the infant. The head-banging is often accompanied by vigorous crib-rocking, and parents have repeatedly reported that the child would rock in his crib so vigorously that the crib would have to be fixed solidly in place to keep it from banging into the furniture and walls in the child's room.

The parents have typically become quite worried between the fourth and 18th months because by this time most infants have begun to socialize in a number of ways, whereas their child seems to be completely preoccupied with head-banging or fixated upon small toys or other inanimate objects. Ritualistic play with certain objects is a very common symptom and the toys that are given to the child are rarely used in the normal manner. Instead, toys are handled in ways which show that the child has no concept of the true function of the toy. For example, an autistic child, rather than running a toy truck along the ground as normal children do, will hold it in his hand while spinning the wheels for long periods, sometimes for hours. Or the truck may be turned on its top and spun on the floor. The child also spins various other objects, such as pot lids, bottles, ashtrays, and whatever else he can lay his hands on. It is not uncommon for parents to report that their child will spend many hours a day spinning various objects, sometimes keeping several objects spinning in one room while he runs to the next room to spin some more, then rushes back to the first room to keep the first group in motion.

Perhaps the most disturbing of the symptoms of autism that occur in early life is what Kanner has called autistic aloneness. It is this symptom that gave the disorder its name. The child will sit and stare into space for extended periods of time, seemingly in a remote dreamworld. Calling his name or trying to attract his attention in any way is unsuccessful. The child seems very much as though he is lost in thought, although as indicated earlier, this impression is a very misleading consequence of the child's facial resemblance to the adult who is lost in thought. Some of the parents describe their child as being "locked in a glass ball." A Swedish psychologist, Karin Junker, has written a book titled *The Child in the Glass Ball*, which is a biographical account of the life of her own daughter (Junker, 1964).

Most of the children seem to be unaware of or uninterested in people, although there are a number of children who clearly have an aversion to other people rather than being merely uninterested in them.

Feeding problems are almost invariably found in children with autism. Some children will insist on eating only certain foods and will have nothing to do with any other food or drink. One child, who had learned to drink from a transparent container, went without taking liquids for several days until it was discovered that he would drink only from a transparent container. Frequently children with classical autism are extremely neat and tidy in their habits and become very upset at any untidiness. One such child began eating with a spoon at nine months and from that point never spilled food on the table or himself. When his clothes did become soiled in any way, he would scream and fuss until they were changed for clean ones.

A striking characteristic of children with autism is the high frequency of repetitive behavior and fetishlike preoccupation with mechanical objects. It is typical of such children to become very engrossed with certain appliances around the house, such as vacuum cleaners, stoves, or refrigerators. Light switches seem to hold a special attraction for them, as do faucets. The children typically react with a violent temper tantrum when any attempt is made to divert them from these preoccupations.

One of the strongest and most characteristic symptoms of classical infantile autism is what Kanner has termed obsessive insistence upon the preservation of sameness in the environment. This is one of the two symptoms that Kanner has reported as being completely necessary for a diagnosis of autism to be reached. The other symptom is the self-imposed isolation—the "autistic aloneness"—described earlier. Insistence on the preservation of sameness is seen in a multitude of ways in these children. In some cases, the child has been known to scream uncontrollably until it was discovered that an article of furniture had been moved from its usual position and that this was distressing to the child. In other cases, the removal of a picture from a wall has brought on a temper tantrum. Rituals, such as the order in which the child's bedclothes are put on him in the evening prior to his bed time, are also a frequent source of temper tantrums when the sameness of the environment, that is, the ritual, is violated. Another way in which this symptom is manifested might be in the child's insistence that the path taken between his home and another point, for example, a store or a relative's house, be invariably followed when going between those two points. If the mother decides to cross the street to look into a shop window or makes some other diversion from the usual path, the child screams and shows signs of distress until the usual route is again taken.

It is almost universal for parents of autistic children to report their strong suspicion of deafness in the child's first year or two of life. Even though they suspected the child might be deaf, they usually also had good reason to believe the child was not deaf, because he showed many indications of exceedingly acute hearing. For example, he might run to the window to look out after hearing a car door slam that no one else in the room had heard. On the other hand, one might call his name loudly and repeatedly or try to gain his attention in other ways with no success. (Similar instances of apparently "selective" attention are seen in laboratory animals with experimentally induced cerebral lesions.)

Many of the parents, having reported that their early suspicion of deafness had been disconfirmed, have next reported a strong suspicion that the child was mentally retarded. Certainly the children are retarded from the standpoint of being unable to do very many of the things that their age-mates can do, such as speaking meaningfully or following instructions. However, the children with classical autism are readily differentiable from the typical retarded child in many ways. For one, facial appearance is almost invariably that of a very intelligent and attractive child. The ordinary retardate whose retardation is so severe that it is detected in the early years of life is usually afflicted with physical stigmata and/or the dull expression which is so characteristic of the individuals with markedly low IQs.

The children with autism typically have a number of rather striking abilities which distinguish them quite clearly from the retardate. Early use of language is one of these skills, although, as it turns out, the language is not meaningfully employed even though it may be articulated very clearly. Additionally, the child frequently shows great skill at remembering tunes and being able to hum or sing them with perfect pitch. Moreover, the child can frequently do various kinds of puzzles, particularly jigsaw puzzles, with great speed and skill. Surprisingly often, the parents have reported their amazement at finding the child assembling a jigsaw puzzle face down by looking only at the shape of the pieces and paying no attention to the picture. As might be expected from the child's characteristic trait of obsessive insistence upon the preservation of sameness, children with autism tend to have remarkably good memories. Kanner has reported an incident in which a child who was shown a roomful of toys, including a jumble of blocks spread all over the floor, screamed vigorously when one of the blocks on the floor was turned in the several days that elapsed between the child's first and second visit.

The motor and manual ability of autistic children is another striking characteristic. Children with classical autism have been described who have been able to climb to great heights, walk along the top boards of very narrow fences, and perform other feats requiring cat-like agility without ever falling or getting hurt. Manual dexterity is also characteristically good in such children. A number of writers have described cases of autism who at the early age of three were able to balance a dime on edge. One 12-year-old boy who had been taught the numbers on the typewriter was able to type the series to 1000 without making an error at an estimated speed of 60 words per minute.

As is evident from the foregoing description, many children with autism would seem to fall into the realm of idiot savant, about which a great deal has been written in psychological literature. I have made a special study of idiot savant abilities in autistic children (as yet unpublished) and find that indeed idiot savant characteristics of a remarkable sort are far more typical in children with infantile autism than in any other population. On the other hand, there are many cases of idiots savant reported in the literature who are clearly not cases of autism.

Calendar calculation is an ability of the idiot savant sort found in a number of classical cases of autism. Children with this ability are able to answer instantly such questions as, "In which months during the year 1958 did the eighth of the month fall on a Wednesday?" Another such question might be, "In the year 1984, what date will the second Friday in August fall on?" A number of investigators have attempted, with very little success, to understand the mental operations that lead to instant and almost invariably accurate answers to these kinds of questions.

The speech abilities of autistic children are quite remarkable in many ways, although as noted earlier, only about half of all children with Kanner's syndrome are able to use speech. Many parents report that they thought their child was a "budding genius" because of his early use of words. It is not uncommon for a child to begin the use of sentences before his first birthday. Between his seventh and 12th months, one autistic boy exhibited the following vocabulary: mamma, dada, bear, spoon, hungry, done, ball, and "C'mon let's play ball." Sometimes a child who has been speaking for several years will cease to speak for a period of a year or more and then resume speech. In some instances, speech is discontinued and never resumed. Again, it should be understood that when speech is used, it is of a peculiar, uncommunicative sort that in some ways is almost more frustrating to the listener than would be the complete absence of speech.

Kanner has published a number of papers devoted specifically to the children's speaking characteristics, and has given names to a number of these unusual characteristics. One of the most striking speech characteristics of children with classical autism is their failure to use the pronoun "I" until their eighth year or beyond. Instead, they use the word "you." For example a child who wants a cookie might approach his mother and say, "You want a cookie," or "Do you want a cookie?" The substitution of you for I is known as pronominal reversal.

Another word which is absent from the vocabulary of the speaking autistic children until perhaps their eighth year or beyond is the simple word "yes." When an autistic child wants to say "yes," he will typically respond by repeating the question. If you offer a child with Kanner's syndrome a cookie and say, "Do you want a cookie?" he will repeat the question after you, "Do you want a cookie?" thus signifying yes. This characteristic is known as affirmation by repetition. Saying "no" is usually accomplished by merely saying no or by the child using some signal such as grunting and waving his hands.

Another one of the speech characteristics is extreme literalness. An example of extreme literalness given by Kanner is the boy whose father attempted to teach him to say the word yes by carrying the boy on his shoulders. The boy loved to be carried on the father's shoulders and the father naturally enough used this as a reward for teaching the child to speak properly. The child did learn to use the word yes, but only to mean "Yes, I want to be carried on your shoulders." To an autistic child who has learned the word "down" in the context of putting something down on the floor, there is great difficulty in appreciating that you can also put something down on a chair or a table.

Metaphorical use of language is also frequently seen in the speaking autistic child. One boy always used the sentence, "Don't throw the dog off the balcony," to indicate "no." His mother had long before said, "Don't throw the dog off the balcony," to him when she saw him about to throw a toy dog off the balcony in a railroad station. Another example of metaphorical use of language was seen in a seven-year-old boy who used the phrase, "He knocked me down," to indicate any blow, pat, spank, or bump inflicted by a person of either sex, accidentally or deliberately.

Part–whole confusion was another of the speech characteristics identified by Kanner in his original series of papers on autism. One three-year-old autistic boy used the expression, "Do you want some catsup, Honey?" to ask for his favorite food, which was hamburger patty with a small amount of catsup on it. The same child used the expression "Bumped the head," whenever he was hurt, even though it might be an elbow or a knee that had been injured.

One of the most noteworthy speech characteristics of autism is delayed echolalia. In delayed echolalia, the child will simply repeat a phrase or sentence, often out of context and with no apparent purpose. For example, one child for months repeated the sentence, "It's all dark outside," even on bright and sunny days. It is frequently reported that autistic children repeat radio and TV commercials endlessly. The speech tone of the autistic child when engaged in delayed echolalia is very unusual. The voice is described as being a hollow, high-pitched monotone, almost as though a robot were speaking. Many parents of autistic children report that their child will print brand names, slogans, and other things he has seen on TV commercials, in a sort of graphic version of delayed echolalia.

Prognosis in autism has been found to be closely linked to the speaking ability of the children. The follow-up study of the first 63 autistic children seen by Kanner reported that 32 had developed speech that was at least somewhat useful and communicative by the age of five. Of these 32 children, 16 were able to achieve *fair* to *good* social adjustment. Of the remaining 31 nonspeaking children, only one even reached a *fair* level. All three of the children whose outcome was described as *good,* as well as 16 of those 46 described as *poor,* came from the speaking group. Of the first 63 children, 34 had been institution-alized at the time of this follow-up study, which was conducted when the median age of the children was 15. The long-term prognosis of children with classical autism has not been good, even though it is somewhat better for the speaking than for the nonspeaking children. Among Kanner's earliest cases, a few seemed to have recovered completely or almost completely and were getting along rather well. One recovered autistic child, for example, became a mathematician, having completed his undergraduate training in mathematics in three years at one of the nation's foremost universities. Another became a meteorologist and composer. However, such favorable outcomes have been reported in only the minority of cases. A fascinating parents-eye report of near-recovery appears in the book *For The Love of Ann* (Copeland, 1973).

THE PARENTS OF AUTISTIC CHILDREN

One of the major controversies surrounding Kanner's original reports on autism concerned his finding extraordinarily high levels of intellectual ability and achievement among the parents of the children who fit the unique symptom pattern he had termed early infantile autism. In his original article, Kanner provided the following description of the parents of his first eleven cases:

Four fathers are psychiatrists, one is a brilliant lawyer, one a chemist and law school graduate employed in the Government Patent Office, one a plant pathologist, one a professor of forestry, one an advertising copy writer who has a degree in law and has studied in three universities, one is a mining engineer and one a successful business man.

Nine of the eleven mothers are college graduates. Of the two who have only a high school education, one was a secretary in a pathology laboratory, and the other ran a theatrical booking office in New York City before marriage. Among the others, there was a free lance writer, a physician, a psychologist, a graduate nurse, and Frederick's mother was successively a purchasing agent, the director of secretarial studies in a girls school, and a teacher of history.

Among the grandparents and collaterals there are many physicians, scientists, writers, journalists and students of art. All but three of the families are represented either in *Who's Who in America* or in *American Men of Science* or in both [1943, p. 248].

A few years later, in 1949, Kanner was able to report his findings on the parents of the first 55 autistic children he had seen. He noted that his "search for unsophisticated parents of autistic children had remained unsuccessful to date." In 1954 he reported on the first 100 sets of parents:

Fathers: Ninety-six were high school graduates, (two of the non-graduates were immigrants). Eighty-seven entered college, 74 graduated college, 38 did postgraduate work. Thirty-one were business men, 12 engineers, 11 physicians (including five psychiatrists), 10 lawyers, 8 tradesmen, 5 chemists, 5 military officers, 4 writers, 3 Ph.D.'s in science, 2 Ph.D's in humanities, 2 teachers, 2 rabbis, and one each: psychologist, dentist, publisher, professor of forestry, and photographer.

Mothers: Ninety-two high school graduates, 70 of whom entered college; 49 graduated; 11 did postgraduate work. Seventeen were secretaries, 16 teachers, 6 business women, 6 librarians, 4 artists, 4 social workers, 3 writers, 3 nurses, 3 telephone operators, 2 psychologists; and one each: physician, lawyer, chemist, Ph.D. in humanities, physiotherapist and laboratory technician.

In addition to observing the very high levels of educational achievement of the parents, Kanner also noted that they had as a group a rather distinctive personality pattern. They were described as cold, bookish, formal, introverted, rather humorless and detached, and even excessively rational and objective:

Nevertheless, aside from the indisputably high level of intelligence, the vast majority of the parents of autistic children have features in common which it would be impossible to disregard. . . .

Most of the parents declare outright that they are not comfortable in the company of people; they prefer reading, writing, painting, making music, or just "thinking." Those who speak of themselves as sociable tend to qualify this by explaining that they have no use for ordinary chatter. They are, on the whole, polite and dignified people who are impressed by seriousness and disdainful of anything that smacks of frivolity [Kanner, 1949, p. 421].

The rate of mental illness among the parents and blood relatives of Kanner's first 100 autistic cases was strikingly low, being only 13 out of 973 parents, grandparents, aunts and uncles. This is about one-third the rate of mental illness in the general population.

Needless to say, these findings set off a great deal of controversy. In the first place, many people preferred to believe that the high intellectual level reported by Kanner was merely a result of the selective referral of well-to-do people to Kanner's clinic, in the mistaken impression that Kanner tended to see only a relatively high socioeconomic level clientele. Adding to the controversy were the reports of investigators who claimed that they had done research on the intellectual and socioeconomic status of parents of children whom *they* called autistic, and their reports supposedly did not confirm Kanner's findings. For the most part, these contradictory findings were based on groups of children who did not meet Kanner's criteria for autism. My book *Infantile Autism* presents a thorough review of this topic. I took the position, based on a comprehensive study of the world literature, including reports of cases of true autism published prior to 1943 and unknown to Kanner, that Kanner's findings on parent intellectuality were valid. Subsequent research, by myself and others, has borne out this position. These findings are discussed later in the present paper.

Perhaps the most far-reaching controversy that erupted as a result of Kanner's papers on autism was concerned with the possibility that the parents' cold, distant "refrigerator-type" personality may have caused the childrens' disorder, which was at the time widely thought to be functional. Kanner himself stated that he believed the parents' distant personalities had only an indirect bearing on the child's disorder. He was, however, widely misquoted on this point. Again, this part of the controversy is taken up in the next section, dealing with recent research on autism.

The foregoing presentation of the syndrome of autism and of information on parental intelligence and personality is a highly condensed version of this material from Chapters 1 and 2 of my book (Rimland, 1964). The book covers a great deal of information which is quite impossible to deal with in the limited space available here. The topics covered include a cognitive theory of autism, the differentiation of autism from schizophrenia, a neurophysiological theory of cognition and personality in both autism and normals, and a great deal more.

Let us now turn to some of the recent empirical research findings that relate to the topics already mentioned.

RECENT RESEARCH ON AUTISM

Diagnostic Check List Forms E-1 and E-2

The first printing of my book *Infantile Autism* included a diagnostic questionnaire titled Form E-1. Form E-1 consisted of 76 questions on such topics as the child's birth history, symptomatology, speech characteristics, and age of onset of disorder. It was designed to be answered by the parents, and for the responses to be readily entered on punched cards for analysis. Within a week of the publication date I began receiving completed copies of Form E-1. Analyses of the forms and the letters accompanying them made it clear that some revisions were needed. This was expected and desired—it was why I had titled the form *E*, for Experimental.

I made the needed changes and called the revised version Form E-2. Like Form E-1, Form E-2 was intended to provide a quantifiable, *objective* means of diagnosing infantile autism. My publisher was kind enough to let me substitute Form E-2 for Form E-1 in the second and all subsequent printings of *Infantile Autism*. Form E-2 has been reproduced by the thousands and widely distributed. The remainder of this paper deals primarily with findings from Form E-2.

The most serious deficiency of the earlier version Form E-1 is worth noting, however. The instructions indicated the form was intended for children up to about age seven, but the replies from parents made it very clear that seven was too late—dramatic and sudden behavioral changes had occurred long before this, and the changes were clearly such as to obscure the diagnosis. Study of the E-1 forms and case histories then at hand led me to conclude that psychotic children very commonly showed striking changes in their behavior patterns at age five and a half. The changes came about quite suddenly and were entirely unexpected. Many of the symptoms of autism faded away before the sixth birthday. Form E-2 was therefore written to obtain information about the child's behavior *prior* to age five.

While I regard these large and fortuitously discovered behavioral changes at age five and a half as being of considerable theoretical importance, I cannot go into the matter in any detail here. I have discussed the matter elsewhere (Rimland, 1968) and am still investigating it. My main reason for bringing up the matter of age five and a half now is to point out that I believe the failure to appreciate the discontinuity of behavior in autistic and autistic-type children after age five has contributed greatly to the present confusion regarding the diagnosis of these children.

There are two other matters I would like to discuss briefly before going on to the analysis of Form E-2.

Autistic Children Versus Autistic-Type Children

The discussion below deals largely with the use of Form E-2 as a means of identifying classical infantile autism. There are good reasons for singling out true autism as the first target of research, but it should not be thought that children with nonautistic childhood psychoses are any less important or are being neglected. As seen below, our research is also aimed at clarifying the murky diagnostic picture as it pertains to these other children as well.

Validity of Parent Reports

The use of a parent-completed questionnaire has been criticized by some, because earlier studies have tended to show that retrospective reports by parents were rather unreliable. Instead, it is suggested, one must actually see the child in one's own office to be confident of a diagnosis. There are many reasons for disagreeing with this position. For one, since diagnosis depends at least in part on retrospective information (e.g., age of onset and behavior in infancy or before age five), there is no way of circumventing parental reports in any case. Even behaviors the child may be manifesting currently may not be seen in the diagnosticians's office or at any other predetermined time and place of observation. Additionally, the studies to be reported below show that Form E-2 does in fact yield highly useful information consistent with laboratory and other types of data. This may be in part a result of the atypicality of the children assessed with Form E-2—because these are sick children, the parents tend to pay close attention to them, and to have repeated their stories again and again to various professionals. Finally, the record of diagnostic reliability and validity in psychiatry, even when the diagnostician has had ample opportunity to see the patient first hand, is anything but encouraging. Given my choice between having a completed Form E-2 or an opportunity to see the child and talk to the parents, I would, so far as research diagnosis is concerned, vastly prefer to have Form E-2.

THE FORM E-2 DATA BANK

Since 1965, when the Diagnostic Check List for Behavior-Disturbed Children, Form E-2, became available, completed forms have been sent to me by parents and professionals from around the world. As of this writing, our files contain over 4000 completed E-2 forms. We have forms from every state in the United States and from 30 foreign countries, including not only the large countries such as England, Germany and Italy, but also Finland, Israel, Kenya, New Zealand, Lebanon, and Switzerland. We also have cases from several Communist Bloc countries: Yugoslavia, Poland, and Czechoslovakia.

Most of our cases have been submitted directly by the parents, but many others have been sent to us by the several hundred professionals with whom we collaborate.

The most recent analysis of our data covered 2218 cases. Of these 1652 (74.5%) are boys and 566 (25.5%) are girls.

Form E-2 consists of 80 questions to be answered by the parents. These questions provide for a detailed description of the child's case from birth through age five. The questions cover not only all of the speech and behavior symptoms mentioned by Kanner in his descriptions of classical autism, but also most of the characteristics (such as clinging and whirling) mentioned by others such as Despert and Bender in their case studies of "symbiotic psychosis" and "childhood schizophrenia." Also included are questions gleaned from the reading of hundreds of letters and reports from parents.

To determine if a child is a true case of autism, Form E-2 is "scored" as though it were a test. One + point is accrued for each question (sign or symptom) characteristic of classical autism, and one − point is scored for each question answered in the nonautistic (schizophrenic?) direction. The child's total "autism" score is the difference between his autism (+) and nonautism (−) scores.

In the absence of a substantial number of cases diagnosed through the use of laboratory tests, there is no completely adequate technology for developing a perfect scoring key for Form E-2, and thus the keys described below must be considered only approximations. On the other hand, as seen, some very good results have been achieved with the E-2 keys.

The most recently derived scoring key for Form E-2 (March 1971) provides a score range of −42 to +45, based on the then-available sample of 2218 cases. I regard a score of +20 or higher as highly indicative of classical early infantile autism. A score of +20 means that the child exhibits at least 20 more signs of classical autism than signs of nonautism.

The cutting score of +20 was set in 1965, after careful analysis of all Form E-2 data and all other data available for the total sample of 68 children then available. The cutting score of +20 was set (albeit tentatively) despite the fact that 25 cases of the 68 (37%) had scored higher than +20, and I was of course well aware from both Kanner's estimate and my own work that a much smaller proportion of the population should be classified as having true autism. I had to assume that classical autism was overrepresented in my early cases. My judgment as to where the cutting score should be set has been supported by later events, as noted below. As the number of E-2 forms at hand grew larger, the present value of 9.7% was reached. This is very close to Kanner's 10% estimate of the occurrence of classical autism in a population of psychotic children.

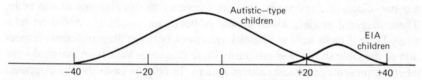

Figure 1.   Frequency distribution of total autism scores as derived from Form E-2. Overlapping curves depict hypothetical separation of true autistic cases from distribution of scores of autistic-type children.

Figure 1 shows my representation of the theoretical relationship between the E-2 scores and the actual occurrence of infantile autism. The small curve to the right shows the distribution of E-2 scores I believe would be found in a population diagnosed with great accuracy through the use of a blood, urine, tissue culture, or other laboratory test, if available. A certain proportion of the true cases would be expected to fall below the +20 cutting score (these are false negatives) while a smaller proportion of nontrue cases would be expected to score above a +20 (false positives). The +20 score is thus a conservative cutting score—for purposes of research it is far better to misdiagnose true cases than to misdiagnose false cases. (Better yet would be never to misdiagnose at all, but that is beyond the state of the art, even for such better-understood conditions as tuberculosis and pregnancy.)

In soliciting cases we have emphasized that we are interested in receiving completed E-2 forms for children with severe behavior disorders, especially children who have been or might be diagnosed as "autistic," "childhood schizophrenic," or "severely emotionally disturbed." We have tried to exclude cases of retardation, except where there are definite psychotic features. We thus have, intentionally, a wide range of disorders in our sample.

Form E-2 contains a space marked "Diagnosis," where the parent is asked to write in the diagnoses given by the professionals who have seen the child. These write-ins include an enormous range of responses, including "autistic," "psychotic," "atypical," "emotional withdrawal," "mental block," and "hopeless," to cite just a few examples. Table 1 shows the more frequent diagnoses.

How much confidence can one have in the labels assigned? A number of respondents have entered as many as five diagnoses on a single E-2 form, and one parent listed the 10 diagnoses attached to the child by various professionals who had seen him. To see the lack of agreement between diagnosticians who have all seen the same child is to be convinced that the state of the diagnostic art is nothing short of chaotic. To illustrate graphically what is so obvious from inspection of the forms themselves, I have constructed Table 2, using the first 445 E-2 forms on which the eight most common diagnoses were listed twice by the parent. Only the first two diagnoses listed have been counted. Where the two diagnosticians agree, the entry appears in the diagonal of the table. These diagonal entries, which appear in boxes for emphasis, should be relatively large if there were substantial agreement between diagnosticians. Inspection of the table shows how arbitrarily these diagnoses have been assigned—the labelling presents an almost random pattern. In only 61 cases did the diagnoses agree. A child called autistic or said to have infantile autism by the first diagnostician has less than one chance in four of being so diagnosed by the second. Clearly, there is a compelling need for a more adequate way of arriving at diagnoses if meaningful scientific work on the cause and cure of the childhood psychoses is to be accomplished. Form E-2 was developed to fill this void.

THE VALIDITY OF THE FORM E-2 AUTISM SCORE

Since clinical diagnoses of children with severe behavior disorders clearly have little value, what reasons are there for believing that Form E-2 can improve the situation? There are several reasons.

Construct Validity

By comparing the responses of true cases of autism (having E-2 scores above +20) with those of children who are psychotic but not autistic (autistic-type

Table 1.   Diagnoses Reported for 2,218 Psychotic Children

Diagnosis	N	Percent
Autistic	651	29.4
Infantile autism or early infantile autism	168	7.6
Childhood schizophrenia	119	5.4
Emotionally disturbed or mentally ill	134	6.0
Brain damaged or neurologically damaged	163	7.3
Retarded	189	8.5
Psychotic or symbiotic psychosis	43	1.9
Deaf or partly deaf	16	.7
Miscellaneous	735	33.2
Total	2218	100.0

children), it is evident that the high-scoring children manifest the syndrome that Kanner described. This is illustrated in Table 3 by means of data from several sample items taken from an item analysis of Form E-2. The item analysis was performed to ensure that all the items in the scoring key were discriminating properly between the autistic and autistic-type children. To maximize the discriminating power of the key, only a small group of 118 especially high-scoring autistic cases was used, and these were divided into speaking $(N = 65)$ and essentially nonspeaking $(N = 53)$ subgroups. For comparison purposes a large group $(N = 230)$ of autistic-type children was chosen from the middle of the E-2 range (scores of -10 to $+5$).

While some of the nonautistic children present a number of symptoms of autism, the true cases always show a marked preponderance of the key symptoms. The items most descriptive of autism, as delineated by Kanner, show very large percentage differences favoring the true autistic group.*

Agreement with Diagnoses of Some of Kanner's Patients

Among the first 2218 cases analyzed were 31 children whose parents indicated that their child had been diagnosed by Leo Kanner. Twenty-two of the 31 reported the diagnosis to have been "autism" or "infantile autism," while eight reported such nonautistic diagnoses as "retarded," and "schizophrenic." One child, with an E-2 score of $+33$, was said to have been diagnosed as "autistically remote." This child was deleted from the analysis.

It must be recognized at the outset that there might very well be inaccuracies in these records. Nevertheless, as a matter of interest, the mean E-2 autism score was computed for each group and the significance of the difference deter-

*There is a minor statistical artifact here in that the items themselves were used in defining the key development groups, but the differences observed are so large that correcting the percentages for redundancy would clearly have little or no effect on the findings reported.

Table 2. Agreement between Pairs of Diagnosticians on the Diagnoses Assigned to 445 Children Showing Severe Behavior Disorders

First Diagnosis	Second Diagnosis								
	Autistic	Infantile Autism or Early Infantile Autism	Childhood Schizophrenia	Emotionally Disturbed or Mentally Ill	Brain Damaged, Neurologically Damaged	Retarded	Psychotic (Symbiotic Psychosis), etc.	Deaf or Partly Deaf	Total
Autistic	33	5	53	18	23	51	10	7	200
Infantile autism or early infantile autism	1	10	6	–	4	6	–	2	29
Childhood schizophrenia	17	3	1	2	8	1	–	–	32
Emotionally disturbed or mentally ill	12	2	4	2	9	13	3	–	45
Brain damaged or neurologically damaged	14	3	2	5	4	15	–	1	44
Retarded	21	2	6	18	16	5	2	2	72
Psychotic (symbiotic psychosis), etc.	4	–	1	1	2	2	–	–	10
Deaf or partly deaf	4	1	–	2	–	5	1	–	13
Total	106	26	73	48	66	98	16	12	445

Table 3. Sample Items from Form E-2 and Response Percentages from Groups of Autistic and Autistic-Type Children

	Autistic[a]		Non-autistic[a]	
Item	Speaking (N = 65)	Mute (N = 53)	(N = 230)	Key
21. Did you ever suspect the child was very nearly deaf?				
___ 1 Yes	77	94	54	(+)
___ 2 No	23	6	46	(−)
	100	100	100	
29. (Age 2-5) Is he cuddly?				
___ 1 Definitely, likes to cling to adults	2	2	20	(−)
___ 2 Above average (likes to be held)	8	8	18	(−)
___ 3 No, rather stiff and awkward to hold	90	88	56	(+)
___ 4 Don't know	0	2	6	
	100	100	100	
33. (Age 3-5) How skillful is the child in doing fine work with his fingers or playing with small objects?				
___ 1 Exceptionally skillful	71	75	33	(+)
___ 2 Average for age	6	9	23	(−)
___ 3 A little awkward, or very awkward	15	8	33	(−)
___ 4 Don't know	8	8	11	
	100	100	100	
40. (Age 3-5) How interested is the child in mechanical objects such as the stove or vacuum cleaner?				
___ 1 Little or no interest	19	9	23	(−)
___ 2 Average interest	4	0	21	(−)
___ 3 Fascinated by certain mechanical things	77	92	56	(+)
	100	100	100	
45. (Age 3-5) Does child get very upset if certain things he is used to are changed (like furniture or toy arrangement, or certain doors which must be left open or shut)?				
___ 1 No	4	2	29	(−)
___ 2 Yes, definitely	87	86	41	(+)
___ 3 Slightly true	9	12	30	(−)
	100	100	100	
71. (Age 3-5) Does the child typically say "Yes" by repeating the same question he has been asked? (Example: You ask "Shall we go for a walk, Honey?" and he indicates he does want to by saying "Shall we go for a walk, Honey?" or "Shall we go for a walk?")				
___ 1 Yes, definitely, does not say "yes" directly	94	12[b]	22	(+)
___ 2 No, would say "Yes" or "OK" or similar answer	0	3	8	
___ 3 Not sure	4	6	8	
___ 4 Too little speech to say	2	79	62	
	100	100	100	

[a]All values are expressed as percentages.
[b]A speech item not applicable to the mute group.

155

mined. The 22 cases reportedly called autistic by Kanner showed a mean score of 13.23, while the eight nonautistics had a mean of −2.88. The difference is significant well beyond the .001 level. Thus the E-2 score correlates very strongly with diagnosis by Kanner.

On the other hand, the mean of the supposedly Kanner-diagnosed cases does not reach our minimum score of +20, possibly for some of the following reasons: *(a)* Our criterion of +20 is intentionally conservative, since we are more interested in rejecting false positives than in finding all true positives. *(b)* The aforementioned possibility of inaccurate reporting by the respondents. A child of whom Kanner remarked "autistic symptoms" could innocently be mislabeled "autistic" by the parents. *(c)* The existence in the sample of a substantial number of children who exhibit the speech pattern of true autistic children while not manifesting the behavioral syndrome. This is an interesting and important point that appears not to have been discussed before. This matter is discussed further below.

Agreement with Laboratory Findings

The "payoff" for a paper-and-pencil method of diagnosis resides in its ability to identify cases which are *also* differentiable from the remainder of the population through laboratory techniques.

In the past few years several extremely important studies have been published which show clear evidence of a biochemical abnormality in children with classical autism. In the first of these studies (Boullin, Coleman, & O'Brien, 1970), blood samples were studied from six children whose E-2 scores met the criterion of exceeding +20. The blood platelets were drawn, cultured, then saturated in a solution of radioactive serotonin, an important neurotransmitter. On comparing the rate of serotonin binding of the platelets of the autistic children with the binding rate of a control group of normal children, it was found that five of the autistic children, and none of the normals, had an extremely fast rate of efflux of the serotonin. (The sixth autistic child also showed a serotonin abnormality, but of a different type.)

The question then arose, "Is this abnormality characteristic of only classical cases of autism, or is it found in all psychotic children?" A second study was undertaken to answer this question. The second study was done on a completely blind basis. Seven classically autistic children and three psychotic but not classically autistic children were sent to the laboratory where blood was drawn by technicians who did not know the diagnoses. The biochemical analyses were also done on a blind basis. Only after the serotonin efflux rates had been recorded for all ten children was the sealed envelope containing the E-2 scores opened.

The rate of efflux of serotonin from the blood platelets of the children scoring above +20 on E-2 was found to be far higher (in six out of seven tests) than the efflux from children whose E-2 scores ranged between -10 and $+12$ (three out of three tests). Thirteen additional cases have since been tested, and at the present time the agreement between serotonin efflux test and the Form E-2 diagnosis of autism stands at 19 "hits" versus four "misses" ($p < .01$).

These findings clearly support not only the contention that Form E-2 can identify children with classical autism, but also, as a corollary, that autism is indeed a unique clinical entity and not merely a synonym for childhood psychosis. These studies also tell us that the optimal cutoff for a diagnosis of autism lies somewhere between $+13$ and $+20$.

Agreement with Demographic Data

As stated earlier, Kanner had noted in his first paper on autism that the children uniformly came from families of unusual intellectual ability and academic achievement. His later papers supported this finding, and the present writer's review of the world literature (Rimland, 1964) strongly confirmed that Kanner's report of the high intellectual level of the families was due to neither error nor artifact. Although it strains the credulity of most people who hear of it, there can be no doubt that Kanner's assertion concerning parental intelligence was correct, *if the children in question are diagnosed rigorously*.

Even after I made this point emphatically in *Infantile Autism*, many papers and books have been published in which the authors claimed to have refuted Kanner's finding, yet in which they failed to make the crucial distinction between true autism (Kanner's syndrome) and the remaining 90% of the population of psychotic children (e.g., Lowe, 1966; Bettelheim, 1967; Ritvo, Cantwell, Johnson, Clements, Benbrook, Slagle, Kelly, & Ritz, 1971; Allen, DeMyer, Norton, Pontius, & Yang, 1971; Szurek & Berlin, 1973).*

In contrast to the foregoing authors, who assumed autism was merely a synonym for childhood schizophrenia, Lotter (1967), Rimland (1968), and Treffert (1970) attempted to separate their samples of childhood psychotics into true autistics and others on the basis of symptomatology. These three authors reported highly significant differences favoring the parents of the Kanner-type children, using such criteria as educational level, occupational level, and intelligence and vocabulary test scores. This matter is important not only because it demonstrates how confusion in the literature can result from failures in diagnosis, but also because it has implications concerning the genetic basis of autism and promises to shed light on the biology of intelligence (Rimland, 1964).

---

*Levine and Olson (1968) attempted to replicate Kanner's finding objectively, but they used Form E-1, long after it had been superseded by Form E-2, in diagnosing their sample of three psychotic children. Form E-1, as indicated earlier, was not found sufficiently discriminating.

It should be noted that both Lotter and Treffert, while attempting to adhere to Kanner's description of autism, used less rigorous criteria than those recommended by the present writer, as evidenced by the proportion of their groups which they regarded as representing classical autism. Lotter so classified 28% of his sample of 54 children, while Treffert based his analysis on the 25% of his sample of 280 who bore the closest resemblance to Kanner's cases.

The highest 25% of autism scores on Form E-2 would have a score above +7, as compared with the present writer's more conservative preference for a +20 cutoff score. It would be interesting indeed to apply the Boullin, Coleman, and O'Brien 5-HT efflux test to a large number of children in the +7 to +20 E-2 range to determine more exactly where the score should be set.

THE E-2 SPEECH AND BEHAVIOR SCORES

Thus far the E-2 autism scale has been discussed in terms of total score which is in practice obtained by summing a *behavior* score and a *speech* score. In our earlier sample of 2218 cases, the behavior scores ranged from −33 to +37. The speech score range was from −9 to +13.

The behavior items consist of questions on such symptoms as avoidance of people, gazing into space, fascination with mechanical objects, and insistence on sameness. Speech items cover all of the speech characteristics Kanner has identified, such as delayed echolalia, pronominal reversal, metaphorical usage, and extreme literalness. In the case of both the behavior and speech scores, the higher the score, the more symptoms of classical autism in the child. As indicated earlier, symptoms counter-indicating a diagnosis of autism are subtracted from the autism score; thus both positive and negative scores are possible.

The speech score has proven to be intriguing and also, because about half of the true cases of autism are mute, especially troublesome. A child with a speech score of +7 or higher is regarded as manifesting the speech syndrome described by Kanner. Only 286 children of the 2218 (13%) score so highly (Table 4). However, among the 126 children who score +20 or above on the behavior items—thus manifesting Kanner's syndrome behaviorally—41% score above +7 on the speech items. This is clearly not merely a chance relationship. The high degree of association between the speech and behavior patterns shows that it was correct to assert that a unique syndrome—a homogeneous subgroup in terms of behavioral pathology—had been identified. There must be a common underlying cause which accounts for the association between these ostensibly unrelated phenomena. Also strikingly in confirmation of this position is our finding that of the 126 Kanner-type children who scored above +20 on the behavior score, only four (3%) had speech scores of −1 or below. Of the remaining 2092 children, 549 (26%) had speech scores of −1 or below. If Kanner's

Table 4. Relationship between Autistic Speech and Behavior Scores of 2,218 Autistic and Autistic-Type Children

Autistic Speech Score	Autistic Behavior Score				Total	
	Nonautism −33 to +19		Autism +20 to +37			
	N	Percent	N	Percent	N	Percent
+7 or above	234	11	52	41	286	13
0 to +6	1309[a]	63	70[a]	56	1379	62
−1 to −9	549	26	4	3	553	25
Total	2092	100	126	100	2218	100

[a]Mute children are included in the 0 to +6 category.

original observations had not been accurate, or if they had applied only to the original small group of children, we could not have found these large statistical differences in an entirely new sample.

However, our data also tell us something that had not been anticipated previously. The full-blown autistic speech pattern, described as highly characteristic of speaking autistic children, is also found, albeit infrequently, in some disordered children who are *not* classically autistic. The E-2 form for one child with a highly autistic speech score of +8 and an anomalous behavior score of −22 had appeared in the first group of 68 completed E-2 forms (Rimland, 1968, Fig. 2). As more data have accumulated, this unexpected and seemingly isolated case has been joined by a substantial number of others. Among the approximately 1300 children in Table 4 whose autistic behavior score ranges from 0 to −33, there appear 88 with autistic speech scores of +7 or higher. One such child has a behavior score of −13 and a speech score of +12. Another has a behavior score of −28 and a speech score of +9. Thus, although the autistic speech symptoms are, as shown earlier, closely correlated with the diagnosis of autism, the pattern is not unique to autism. It is thus easily possible to misdiagnose a child as autistic if only his speech is taken into account. This unanticipated phenomenon probably accounts for some of the confusion in diagnosis which is so common. Intensive study is planned of the group with anomolously high speech scores.

THE USE OF E-2 IN SYNDROME DETECTION BY COMPUTER

Form E-2 has been used by a number of investigators in a variety of research studies (e.g., Douglas & Sanders, 1968; Judd & Mandell, 1968). A major purpose of Form E-2 is to provide the raw data needed for the cluster analyses which I believe to be the most promising method now available for discovering the other syndromes, in addition to the syndrome of infantile autism, that constitute the childhood psychoses (Rimland, 1968). Until these additional syndromes are detected so that accurately diagnosed children representing them can be studied, the chances for conducting meaningful medical research on psychotic children with other than Kanner's syndrome are small.

In the past we have relied on astute clinicians to notice that certain symptoms were closely associated with each other and that therefore a syndrome was at hand (e.g., Kanner's discovery of Kanner's syndrome). But computers can be programmed to do this task more efficiently, if the appropriate information can be provided to them.

The first cluster analysis of Form E-2 was performed by James Cameron, then a doctoral candidate at the University of California, Berkeley, as his dissertation project (Cameron, 1969). I provided E-2 data on punched cards which he subjected to the BC-TRY method of computer cluster analysis. The state of the cluster analysis art is still fairly primitive. There is no "right way" to find the best subgrouping of children. Just as different humans may each classify an assortment of objects differently, the various computer methods provide differing solutions. Part of Cameron's project involved comparing different clustering methods. This need not concern us. What is important from our standpoint is that the analysis of the E-2 data did provide a number of subgroups of children, and these subgroups had sufficient stability and integrity to give meaningful results. The subgroups Cameron derived showed many statistically significant differences between the groups on variables of etiological importance. (See discussion of Form E-3 below). Thus Form E-2 may be seen to have utility beyond its original purpose of identifying cases of Kanner's syndrome. Actually, progress in the field of cluster analysis is rapid, and Cameron's work has already been superseded by more powerful computer programs, some of which are now being used for further analyses of our E-2 data bank.

FORM E-3

Unlike Forms E-1 and E-2, which were designed for diagnostic purposes, Form E-3 was devised primarily to provide information of importance in determining the causes of the various childhood psychoses. E-3 consists of approximately 250 questions to be answered by the parents. (We send Form E-3 to parents for completion only after they have sent us a completed Form E-2. If we dared to send them both forms at once for completion, we fear we would not hear from them again!)

One series of questions on Form E-3 concerns the mother's pregnancy: Was she given a gamma globulin shot, or an anti-miscarriage shot? (Many mothers have asked me if their child's problem could have been caused by these injections during their fateful pregnancy, since their other children are normal.) Did the mother get dental work done? (This would expose her to possible hazard from either radiation or mercury ingestion.) What drugs did the mother take during pregnancy? (The relation between thalidomide and phocomelia was discovered by a similar questionnaire.) There are many similar questions.

Another series of questions pertains to the parents and relatives: Blood types of parents? Celiac disease in family? Gout in family? Diabetes? Form E-3 also contains many questions not on Form E-2 pertaining to the child's symptoms, on the medications he has taken and their effects, as well as on other matters of interest.

We have about 1400 completed E-3 forms now for children whose E-2 forms are also on file. The E-3 data, like the E-2 data, are recorded on punched cards—six cards per child for E-3. How do we plan to use these data? Suppose, for example, on analyzing Form E-3, that we find 70% of our cases of classical autism to have relatives with celiac disease, as compared with only 20% in the autistic-type children. This could clearly be a valuable research lead. Or suppose that after completing a cluster analysis and comparing the resulting clusters in terms of E-3 answers we find that 80% of the mothers of the cluster A subgroup of children had been given gamma globulin during pregnancy, while only 20% of the mothers of the children in subgroups B through K had been given gamma globulin. This also could provide a valuable lead to prevention or treatment.

Since we are in touch with researchers in many parts of the world, it may be possible to send blood or urine samples, or perhaps the children themselves, as required, to the laboratory of a researcher with a special interest in the kind of problems our analyses turn up.

Or suppose that as a result of a new study, or as a result of our analyses of the "Treatment Effects" section of Form E-3, we find that several children in subgroup G respond especially well to a new drug or to high dosages of a certain vitamin? Our task would be to see to it that the remainder of the group G children had an opportunity to be tried on the new treatment. Studies of these kinds are in progress at the Institute for Child Behavior Research. Findings will be forthcoming in the next few years.

TREATMENT AND PROGNOSIS

The Megavitamin Experiment

I recently conducted an experiment designed to determine whether large quantities of certain of the B-vitamins might be helpful to children with autism and other forms of childhood psychosis. The study has been reported fully, with numerous citations of the literature, in the book *Orthomolecular Psychiatry* (Rimland, 1973), so I present only an overview of it here.

I had become interested in the possibility that mental disorders might be treatable with high dosage levels of vitamins during the mid-1960s, after reading the reports published by psychiatrists Abram Hoffer and Humphry Osmond. Since 1952, Hoffer and Osmond had been treating adult schizophrenics with very high levels of the B-vitamin niacin, or its alternate form niacinamide, and had achieved what they reported to be truly remarkable results. Hoffer and Osmond take the position that schizophrenia is a genetic metabolic disease that causes its victims to require far more niacin than even a good diet could possibly provide. They were using this vitamin (sometimes called vitamin B-3) at levels ranging from 3000 to 18,000 or more milligrams per day. This form of treatment was severely criticized by the psychiatric establishment. After all, the official "minimum daily requirement" for niacin is about 15 milligrams per day!

Several years of study of the scientific literature and of correspondence with physicians and parents who had been experimenting with the vitamin approach led me to believe that Hoffer and Osmond might well be on the right track. The large, orthodox antivitamin group was, as usual, more interested in maintaining the status quo than in exploring new approaches. It was particularly disconcerting to find psychiatrists criticizing the biological approach advocated by Hoffer and Osmond when hundreds of research studies had been published which showed quite clearly that the "talk therapy" methods of treatment preferred by most psychiatrists—psychotherapy and psychoanalysis—were quite ineffective for both children (Levitt, 1963) and adults (Rachman, 1972).

I designed a study in which nearly 200 psychotic children from all parts of the United States and Canada participated, each under the supervision of a physician of the family's choice. Rather than restricting the study to niacin, I used massive amounts of vitamin C, plus three of the B-vitamins; niacin, pyridoxine, and pantothenic acid. The vitamins were given for a three-month period followed by a one-month no-treatment period during which evaluation of behavior continued. Evaluations of the child were made bi-weekly by the child's parents and monthly by his physician, for four months. The study made use of an unusual design in which clusters of children, grouped by a computer in terms of similarity of answers to Form E-2, were compared in their response to treatment. The computer grouped the children *prior* to being given information on their response to treatment. Significant $p < .02$) intercluster differences were found in vitamin effectiveness scores; thus the marked improvement reported in many of the children was not randomly distributed in the group, but was instead related to the child's medical history and symptomatology.

In a previous study, I had compared 14 drugs with each other as evaluated by the parents of the autistic and autistic-type children on whom they had been tried. Some of the drugs were rated as having impaired more children than they helped. The best of the drugs was Mellaril, which was reported to have helped 36.4% of the 277 children on which it was tried, and to have impaired the behavior of only 19.9% of the children. The comparable figures for the 191 children in the vitamin study were 66.5% helped and 3.7% impaired. Thus, using the criterion of parent (and physician) ratings of therapeutic effectiveness, the vitamins were far better than the best of the drugs.

The children "impaired" by the vitamins had grown irritable and showed several other minor side effects which were quickly reversible upon discontinuance of the vitamins. I later learned that these side effects could have been prevented, in most cases, had I been knowledgable enough to have used supplemental minerals, in normal quantities, in addition to the vitamins.

It is important to emphasize that the theory behind the megavitamin approach does not assume that the patient's diet is inadequate, but instead that the patient has an inordinate need, genetic in most instances, for massive quantities of certain vitamins. Nobel Laureate Linus Pauling has established a laboratory to study such approaches to the treatment of mental illness. He has coined the term orthomolecular psychiatry to refer to the concept that mental illness is best treated by finding the optimal concentration of nutrients normally present in the human body. Since 1954, some 15 genetic disorders have been identified which are characterized by the patient's need for massive amounts of particular vitamins. In some instances, the patient needs five or six hundred times the amount of a vitamin considered sufficient for a normal healthy person. A number of cases have been reported in which "autistic" children were found to be excreting abnormal substances in their urine, and in whom the biochemical error could be corrected by giving the child vitamin B-6. Pyridoxine (Vitamin B-6) is the vitamin which is most often implicated in these "genetic vitamin dependencies."

Of special interest to us is the fact that the children with classical autism were among those showing greatest improvement during the vitamin study. These children showed special responsiveness to pyridoxine, as would be predicted from the findings reported earlier in this paper of an abnormality in the blood level of serotonin in these children. Vitamin B-6 plays an important role in the production and metabolism of serotonin. Research to follow-up these findings is continuing.

PSYCHOLOGICAL AND EDUCATIONAL APPROACHES

After his thorough review of 57 studies in which the rate of improvement of children treated with psychotherapy was compared with that of matched, untreated controls, Levitt (1963) stated that the conclusion was "inescapable" that psychotherapy had not been found to facilitate the recovery of children with "emotional" illness. Lewis (1965), covering much the same ground, reached the same conclusion.

Given that psychotherapy (including psychoanalysis) is not an effective way of modifying the behavior of autistic and autistic-type children, are there other psychological approaches which are effective? Yes, indeed. Operant conditioning has proven to be one approach which is often quite effective. Since another contribution to this volume is addressed to the matter of operant conditioning, I make only a few comments on it in passing.

First, I should respond to a question which is almost always asked of me when I lecture: "If you believe that autism and other forms of psychosis in childhood are organically caused, why do you recommend the use of a psychologically-based treatment like operant conditioning?" I usually answer this question by referring the audience to the case of Helen Keller who was, of course, blind and deaf from an early age, yet who learned to speak and write, and who became an extremely productive and effective person. I point out that the techniques of training Helen Keller were very similar, if not identical to the ones now employed by the practitioners of behavior modification. While Helen Keller did not regain the use of her eyes or her ears, the behavior modification techniques trained her to use the abilities that she had left to the best advantage.

Another question which is often posed relates to the rather limited goals which seem to be the objective of many programs of operant conditioning. Here again, I find it instructive to invoke the case of Helen Keller: even though the goals her teacher set for her appeared to be quite limited (one of Helen's first lessons was to make a sound like "wah-wah" when she wanted water), the fact should not be overlooked that she made great progress, not only through the accumulation of such small steps, but also because she learned, in the process of learning the small steps, how to deploy her attention in such a way that she could make much larger steps later on (Rimland, 1970, 1972). I know of many instances in which children with autism and similar disorders have made remarkable progress even though the behavior modification approach which was employed in teaching them seemed to be so limited in scope and potential that the effort of teaching the children at first hardly seemed worthwhile.

Perhaps the most important objective which can be reached through the application of behavior modification techniques to autistic-type children involves teaching the child to control his behavior to the point where he can adapt to a structured classroom situation. Many have wondered, as I have, why do some autistic and autistic-type children make much more progress in life than others? Much evidence leads to the conclusion that the children who are fortunate enough to be placed in a highly structured, purposeful school situation seem by and large to have the best long-term prognosis. It should be recognized that the present hard-earned recognition of the importance of the structured classroom environment represents a radical departure from the ideas of the past, when it was felt that an unstructured, permissive situation would be best for the children, who were called emotionally disturbed.

A strong advocate of the structured classroom approach is Carl Fenichel, the noted Director of the League School in Brooklyn. At the convention of the National Society for Autistic Children in 1969, Dr. Fenichel explained how he had entered the field of educating so-called emotionally disturbed children with the conviction that what the child needed was love, affection, and a permissive environment. As time went on, however, he began to appreciate the need for structure:

At the beginning, our school had a relatively unstructured and permissive atmosphere and our children were allowed to ventilate their feelings and drives with a hope that the basic, intrapsychic conflicts could be "worked through." . . . Our children taught us otherwise. We learned that disorganized children need someone to organize their worlds for them . . . that what they needed were teachers who knew how to limit as well as accept them. We soon learned the need for a highly organized and structured program of training and education. . . .

Although it would take us somewhat far afield to explore the matter more thoroughly, it should suffice to say that researchers in the United States, Canada, and Great Britain have all come to the same conclusion regarding the importance of a purposeful, nonpermissive educational program for psychotic children, if those children are to have any hope of reaching a higher level of social adequacy (Rimland, 1970; 1972).

In the past several years, Kanner has published two follow-up reports in which he traces the development of his earlier cases of infantile autism through adolescence into young adulthood. In the first of these papers (Kanner, 1971) he reported his follow-up of the first 11 children he had originally described in 1943. Only two of the children were, according to Kanner, "success stories." One was employed as a bank teller, the other as a duplicating machine operator. For some of the others, ". . . state hospital admission was tantamount to a life sentence." In another recent paper (Kanner, 1972), case histories of nine additional children, selected from the 96 children who had been diagnosed "autistic" at Johns Hopkins prior to 1953, were presented in detail. Again, the "successes" in this group were very few.

It is important to recognize, however, that the early cases of autism were raised during a period when psychotherapeutic methods and permissive approaches were in vogue. I am confident that any similar group of children, subjected to the newer procedures of structured education and behavior modification, would fare better. Even more important, in the long run, are the strides that are being made in the biochemistry laboratory. Progress is slow, but progress is being achieved.

REFERENCES

Allen, J., DeMyer, M. K., Norton, J. A., Pontius, W. & Yang, E. Intellectuality in parents of psychotic, subnormal, and normal children. *Journal of Autism and Childhood Schizophrenia*, 1971, **1**, 311–326.

Bettelheim, B. *The empty fortress*. New York: The Free Press, 1967.

Boullin, D. J., Coleman, M., & O'Brien, R. A. Abnormalities in platelet 5-hydroxytryptamine efflux in patients with infantile autism. *Nature*, 1970, **226**, 371–372.

Boullin, D. J., Coleman, M., O'Brien, R. A., & Rimland, B. Laboratory predictions of infantile autism, based on 5-hydroxytryptamine efflux from platelets, and their correlation with the Rimland E-2 scores. *Journal of Autism and Childhood Schizophrenia*, 1971, **1**, 63–71.

Cameron, J. R. Background factors related to various forms of childhood autism. Ph.D dissertation. University of California, Berkeley, 1969.

Copeland, J. *For The Love of Ann*. New York: Ballantine Books, 1973.

Douglas, V. I., & Sanders, F. A. A pilot study of Rimland's Diagnostic Check List with autistic and mentally retarded children. *Journal of Child Psychology and Psychiatry*, 1968, **9**, 105–108.

Ekstein, R. *The challenge: Despair and hope in the conquest of inner space*. Los Angeles, Reiss-Davis Child Center Publication, 1971.

Himwich, H. E., Jenkins, R. L., Fujimori, M., Narasimhachari, N., & Ebersole, M. A biochemical study of early infantile autism. *Journal of Autism and Childhood Schizophrenia*, 1972, **2**, 114–126.

Judd, L. J., & Mandell, A. J. Chromosome studies in early infantile autism. *Archives of General Psychiatry*, 1968, **18**, 450–457.

Junker, K. S. *The child in the glass ball*. Nashville: Abingdon Press, 1964.

Kanner, L. Autistic disturbances of affective contact. *Nervous Child*, 1943, **2**, 217–250.

Kanner, L. The specificity of early infantile autism. *Zeitschrift fur Kinderpsychiatrie*, 1958, **25**, 108–113.

Kanner, L. Follow-up study of eleven autistic children originally reported in 1943. *Journal of Autism and Childhood Schizophrenia*, 1971, **1**, 119–145.

Kanner, L., Rodriguez, A., & Ashenden, B. How far can autistic children go in matters of social adapation? *Journal of Autism and Childhood Schizophrenia*, 1972, **2**, 9–33.

Kanner, L. *Childhood psychosis: Initial studies and new insights*. Washington: Winston & Sons, 1973.

Levine, M., & Olson, R. P. Intelligence of parents of autistic children. *Journal of Abnormal Psychology*, 1968, **73**, 215–217.

Levitt, E. E. Psychotherapy with children: A further evaluation. *Behavior Research and Therapy*, 1963, **1**, 45–51.

Lewis, W. W. Continuity and intervention in emotional disturbance: A review. *Exceptional Children*, 1965, **31**, 465–475.

Lotter, V. Epidemiology of autistic conditions in young children. II. Some characteristics of the parents and children. *Social Psychiatry*, 1967, **1**, 163–173.

Lowe, L. H. Families with early childhood schizophrenia: Selected demographic information. *Archives of General Psychiatry*, 1966, **14**, 26–30.

Rachman, S. *The effects of psychotherapy*. London: Pergamon Press, 1971.

Rimland, B. *Infantile autism*. New York: Appleton-Century-Crofts, 1964.

Rimland, B. On the objective diagnosis of infantile autism. *Acta Paedopsychiatrica*, 1968, **35**, 146–161.

Rimland, B. Freud is dead: New directions in the treatment of mentally ill children. *Distinguished lecture series in special education*. University of Southern California, 1970. Pp. 33–48.

Rimland, B. The differentiation of childhood psychoses: An analysis of checklists for 2,218 psychotic children. *Journal of Autism and Childhood Schizophrenia*, 1971, **1**, 161–174.

Rimland, B. Operant conditioning: Breakthrough in the treatment of mentally ill children. In E. P. Trapp & P. Himelstein (Eds.), *Readings on the exceptional child*. (2nd ed.) New York: Appleton-Century-Crofts, 1972.

Rimland, B. The effect of high dosage levels of certain vitamins on the behavior of children with severe mental disorders. In D. R. Hawkins & L. Pauling (Eds.), *Orthomolecular psychiatry*. San Francisco: W. H. Freeman, 1973.

Ritvo, E. R., Yuwiler, A., Geller, E., Ornitz, E. M., Saeger, K., & Plotkin, S. Increased blood serotonin and platelets in early infantile autism. *Archives of General Psychiatry*, 1970, **23**, 566–572.

Ritvo, E. R., Cantwell, D. Johnson, E., & Clements, M. Social class factors in autism. *Journal of Autism and Childhood Schizophrenia*, 1971, **1**, 297-310.

Szurek, S. A., & I. N. Berlin (Eds.) *Clinical studies in childhood psychoses*. New York: Brunner/Mazel, 1973.

Treffert, D. A. Epidemiology of infantile autism. *Archives of General Psychiatry*, 1970, **22**, 431–438.

Tustin, F. *Autism and Childhood Psychosis*. New York: Science House, 1972.

CHAPTER 5

Research and Treatment with Autistic
Children in a Program of Behavior Therapy

JUDITH STEVENS-LONG AND O. IVAR LOVAAS

One of the most exciting developments in clinical psychology in recent years has been the emergence of behavior modification. Although experimental research on learning principles dates back to Pavlov and Thorndike, the application of these principles to human problems began in earnest only about 15 years ago. The principles of respondent conditioning were first utilized in the development of systematic desensitization by Wolpe et al. (Wolpe, 1968; Wolpe, 1969), while Allyon and Azrin (1965) first applied instrumental conditioning to the treatment of adult schizophrenics. Since that time, a growing number of researchers have examined the utility of learning theory paradigms for modifying deviant behaviors in children including childhood schizophrenia (Wolf, Risley, & Mees, 1964; Risley & Wolf, 1967; Lovaas, Berberich, Perloff, & Schaeffer, 1966; Lovaas, 1967; Lovaas, Koegal, Simmons, & Stevens-Long, 1973), juvenile delinquency (Thorp & Wetzel, 1969), mental retardation (Thompson & Grabowski, 1972), and classroom behavior (O'Leary & Drabman, 1971). This chapter presents an overview of a project established to examine the applicability of instrumental conditioning or reinforcement theory to childhood schizophrenia.

REINFORCEMENT THEORY AND TREATMENT

To understand the viewpoint presented here, one must understand how deviant behavior may be seen from a reinforcement theory framework. In a very simplified way, the development of deviant behavior may be approached with the notion in mind that such behaviors may have come about because of their consequences. That is, as a result of their consequences, they may have been strengthened or weakened. Behaviors are strengthened or weakened as a result

169

of their interaction with positive and negative reinforcing stimuli or, popularly speaking, because of gratification and punishment. Both positive and negative reinforcers can be classified in another way, as primary or secondary reinforcers. Certain stimuli, like food and pain, are called primary reinforcers and appear to have reinforcing properties from the moment of birth. Other stimuli, such as personal closeness and approval, acquire their reinforcing value as the child develops, probably through association with already powerful stimuli. As the child develops, these secondary reinforcers increase vastly in number and variety and come to regulate and control many behaviors typically considered distinctively human, such as interpersonal and intellectual behaviors. Secondary reinforcers are sometimes referred to as learned or conditioned reinforcers, and, after the first few months of life, they are essential to behavioral development and control.

Several authors have argued, for different reasons, that schizophrenic or autistic children fail to develop normally because they fail to acquire secondary reinforcers (Ferster, 1961; Rimland, 1964). If a child were to completely fail to acquire secondary reinforcers, the child should display little, if any, social behavior. It is apparent that such failure need not be complete. Even partial failure to acquire such reinforcers may be predictive of important deficits in social behavior.

The treatment of autism from a reinforcement theory framework could proceed by building behaviors directly, or by establishing secondary reinforcers. In the long run, it may be more therapeutic to attempt to establish secondary reinforcers. However, at the present, we do not know how to build such reinforcers, so we are forced to rely on the use of primary ones, at least in the beginning.

PATIENTS

Most of our research has dealt exclusively with those psychotic children who are sufficiently deficient in emotional, social, and intellectual development to be labeled autistic. We have treated a total of 20 children intensively, all of whom have been diagnosed as autistic by at least one other agency not associated with the project. The majority of the children have been given more than one diagnosis, usually including retarded or brain damaged. Most of the children had been rejected from one or more schools for the emotionally ill or the retarded because their teachers could not control them and because their behavior was so bizarre that it was disruptive for other children in the class.

Clinically speaking, with three or four exceptions, these children seem devoid of anxiety, and none had any awareness that something was wrong with him.

They represented the more underdeveloped or behaviorally regressed of psychotic children.

All of these children exhibit behavioral deficits, but they also have other common problems. Generally, the children can be described along the following dimensions: (1) *Apparent sensory deficit,* this category reflects the fact that when asked to complete the Rimland Diagnostic Checklist for Behavior-Disturbed Children (Rimland, 1964), most of the parents report that their children at one time appeared to be deaf and seemed to look through or walk through things as if they were not there. (2) *Severe affect isolation* was predominant, meaning that the parents indicated on the Rimland Checklist that their children *(a)* fail to reach out to be picked up when approached by other people; *(b)* look at or walk through people as if they weren't there; *(c)* appear so distant that no one can reach them; *(d)* are indifferent to being liked; and *(e)* are not affectionate. (3) Our sample exhibited a high rate of *self-stimulatory behavior,* that is, behavior that appears solely to provide the children with proprioceptive feedback (e.g., rocking, spinning, twirling, flapping, and gazing, (4) *Mutism* occurred in about half of the children in our sample. These children produced no recognizable words. (5) *Echolalic speech* was present in the remaining children. These children echoed the speech of others, either immediately or after a delay, giving the impression of nonrelated inappropriate speech. (6) In all of the children *receptive speech* was minimal or missing all together. Some of the children would obey simple commands, but *all* failed to respond appropriately to more complex demands involving abstract terms such as prepositions, pronouns, and time. (7) There was also an absence of, or only minimal presence of, social and *self-help behaviors:* most of the children could not dress themselves or comb their hair; some of the children were not toilet-trained, and such. (8) Some of these children were self-destructive or *self-mutilatory.* All had severe aggressive tantrumous outbursts, and scratched and bit attending adults when forced to comply with even minimal rules for social conduct.

The problems these children display beside the behavioral deficits may be the cause of the behavioral deficits or their effect, or both may be caused by some third factor. The relationships are not understood. However, some *a priori* decisions can be made about these problems, and they are of sufficient importance to be described here. Let us consider, for example, the problem of self-mutilation. Self-mutilation is most often concurrent with a rage reaction toward a teacher or parent (e.g., kicking, biting, scratching, and punching), less frequently toward physical objects (e.g., turning over tables and chairs, and tearing curtains), and is often accompanied by screaming. It seems pointless to try to teach intellectual behaviors to a child who is chewing off his fingers or banging his head against the concrete. In general, teachers are very upset by a child who self-mutilates, so they avoid such children. Moreover, many of these children are very aggressive toward their teachers, making the teachers panic over the possibility of being bitten or hurt. Thus we decided to try to remove these interfering behaviors.

SELF-DESTRUCTIVE BEHAVIOR

Self-destructive behavior consists primarily of "head-banging" (against walls, floors, furniture, etc.), "arm-banging" (against sharp corners), beating oneself on the head or face with fists or knees, and biting oneself on wrists, arms, and shoulders. Frequently, the behavior is so severe it becomes a major safety problem and the child must be physically restrained by a camisole ("straightjacket") or tied to a bed. The necessity for restraining the child engenders further curtailment of growth, psychological and otherwise, plus anxiety and demoralization in those who care for the child. At one time or another in their lives, a significant number of children who are diagnosed as psychotic or mentally retarded exhibit self-destructive behavior. Traditional treatment usually combines drug and some form of supportive, interpersonal therapy. No evidence demonstrates the effectiveness of any such traditional therapy.

An early paper (Lovaas, Freitag, Gold, & Kassorla, 1965) demonstrated that self-destructive behavior might be adequately conceptualized as learned, social behavior; that is, behavior which is acquired and maintained by social reinforcement (e.g., attention from an adult). Acting upon the implications of this early study, Lovaas and Simmons (1969) attempted to isolate some of the environmental conditions that controlled self-destructive behavior in three severely retarded and psychotic children. We review this paper in some detail.

Three experimental treatment conditions were constructed: two were designed to test conditions under which it was hypothesized that self-destructive behavior might decrease; and one was designed to test some ideas about the conditions under which one might expect the behavior to increase. All three conditions were based upon the assumption that self-destructive behavior is learned, social behavior. The three conditions are outlined below.

1. *Extinction.* If self-destructive behavior is maintained by socially reinforcing consequences, then removing those consequences should weaken and eventually stop the behavior; that is, the behavior should extinguish. Accordingly, two of the children were placed in a small room for 1½ hours in the morning on consecutive days. They were left free to hit themselves. No consequences, social or otherwise, were provided. The third child did not undergo this condition because she had already damaged her ears and eyes quite severely, which prevented leaving her unrestrained. Both children who experienced this condition exhibited a gradual extinction of self-destructive behavior. The

highest response frequency recorded for the first child was 2750 self-destructive acts during the first session. This peak was followed by a gradual reduction to zero by the 10th session. The second child emitted 900 self-destructive acts in the first session. Some 45 sessions later, his rate had decreased to approximately 30 acts per session.

One may conclude from such data that extinction may be an effective procedure for decreasing the frequency of self-destructive acts. Obviously, however, it is not an ideal form of treatment because of the high frequency of self-destructive behavior the child will emit, particularly during the early stages of the procedure. Also, the extinction produced in the study seemed highly situational. It did not generalize beyond the experimental situation. The frequency of self-destructive behavior might be quite low in the room where the experimental extinction had taken place, but might reappear at much higher rates in different rooms, with new people, and so on. These were some of the reasons why the authors sought to suppress the behavior through the use of aversive stimuli.

2. *Aversive stimulation.* Aversive stimulation, that is, punishment, in the form of a one-second shock, was applied to the child's leg as soon as he hit himself. The shock was strong enough to be considered highly aversive by the investigators who tried it on themselves, but it was not strong enough to cause any tissue damage. The shock was delivered using a hand-held inductorium powered by five 1.5-V flashlight batteries. The results of this intervention indicated that the use of shock, contingent upon self-destructive behavior, brings about an immediate suppression of that behavior.

However, as with the extinction procedure, the effect of shock appears to be limited to those situations in which it is administered. If a child is shocked in one room and not another, or by one person and not another, the child will sometimes form a discrimination between these situations. One final aspect of the data should be mentioned. There was some evidence that the side effects of punishment, instead of being undesirable, were positive. The children gave evidence of becoming more affectionate and prosocial following the use of shock.

3. *Worsening self-destructive behavior.* The authors reported several interventions designed to discover what conditions might make self-destructive behavior worse. For example, deprivation and satiation for social reinforcers, that is, social isolation and continual attention, were examined, but neither of these conditions appeared to effect the frequency of self-destructive behavior. However, it was observed that self-destruction increased in strength when we gave sympathetic comments contingent upon the child hurting himself, and that the frequency of the behavior returned to base-line levels when these comments were no longer administered.

It can be concluded that both extinction and punishment are effective in terminating self-destructive behavior. Extinction has the disadvantage that it is not immediately effective and temporarily exposes the child to the danger of severe damage from his own self-destructiveness. Both kinds of interventions appear to be situation specific and must be repeated in many different situations if one wishes to obtain generalization. The data also suggest that the child will revert to self-destruction after treatment is terminated unless conditions in the post-treatment environment are made consistent with the treatment environment.

SELF-STIMULATORY BEHAVIOR

We have also explored in some detail another of the deviant behaviors that is characteristically displayed by autistic children. We refer to this behavior as "self-stimulatory behavior." This category of behavior includes any behavior which seems to serve no other function than to provide the child with sensory input. It takes the form of rocking, spinning, flapping the arms, fondling of self, spinning or twirling objects, crossing or rolling the eyes, gazing and grimacing, and such. For some time, our observations have suggested that self-stimulatory behavior is incompatible with the occurrence of other behaviors (Lovaas et al., 1966). Other investigators have reported the same impression (Risley, 1968). When the autistic child is not paying attention, he appears to be largely engaged in self-stimulatory behavior. In the sense that it appears to be incompatible with attention to a teacher and other more appropriate behaviors, self-stimulation is disruptive to any attempts at treatment.

These observations suggested to us that self-stimulation may form a basis for the "unresponsiveness" and withdrawal that so many investigators consider to be the major stumbling block to the treatment of autistic children. Kanner and Eisenberg (1957) and Rimland (1964) among others have provided more extensive clinical descriptions of the problem of "unresponsiveness." Hermelin and O'Connor (1966) provide illustrations of more systematic assessment of the children's unresponsiveness.

It is possible that self-stimulation produces a decreased level of arousal in the child, even a sleep-like state. Brackbill, Adams, Crowell, and Gray (1966), working with normal children, and Stone (1964), have both presented data that show that continuous, monotonous stimulation may produce a decreased level of arousal. With this in mind, we undertook an empirical study designed to assess whether self-stimulation was related to inattention (Lovaas, Litrownik, & Mann, 1971).

Twelve children participated in the 1971 study. Eight of the children had been diagnosed autistic (four were mute and four were echolalic). The remaining four children were normal. The echolalic autistics were functioning at a slightly higher level than the mute children; that is, the echolalic children used some speech and exhibited more appropriate social and self-help behaviors.

The children were placed in an experimental room that was bare, except for a chair and a candy dispenser. The experimenter could observe the child from an adjoining room through a one-way mirror. The experimenter trained the children to respond to a tone by getting up from the chair, walking five feet to the M and M candy dispenser, retrieving a piece of candy, and returning to the chair. A timer was automatically activated when the tone sounded and stopped automatically when the child left the chair. The timer thus provided a measure of the child's response latency, showing how long it took the child to respond to the tone.

After the children had learned to get up and retrieve the candy when the tone came on, we began a series of experimental observations. Two observers watched the children, noting whether the child was engaged in self-stimulatory behavior at the onset of the tone. Integration of these observations with response latencies showed that normal and echolalic children were equally responsive, but the mute children showed longer and more variable response latencies when they were engaged in self-stimulatory behavior. However, the data also demonstrate that the latencies of these mute children decreased over successive sessions. It appeared that the mute autistics were gradually learning to overcome the blocking effect that seemed to be associated with self-stimulation.

Subsequent experimental work led to several other significant observations about self-stimulatory behavior. It was demonstrated that the amount of self-stimulation varied with deprivation for extrinsic (food) reinforcers. If the children were given as many M and M's as they wanted before entering the experimental room, the amount of self-stimulation increased significantly. Other observations demonstrated that the children displayed significantly less self-stimulation in the experimental room than in some other neutral room in which they had never experienced any training of appropriate behaviors.

The conclusion drawn from these data, simply stated, was that self-stimulation is maintained by reinforcers which compete with those which maintain other kinds of behaviors. The data suggest that response latencies, or degree of unresponsiveness, may be manipulated by varying the strength of reinforcement for other behaviors.

Our discussion of self-stimulation and self-destruction illustrates research designed primarily to provide guidelines for the analysis of pathological behavior. However, by far the greatest part of our effort has been directed at establishing behavior that the children have failed to acquire. At this point, let us turn to a review and discussion of two programs central to this part of our effort: a program for teaching imitation and one for teaching meaning. This outline is intended to give the reader some insight into the methodology employed and the results obtained. This is by no means a comprehensive survey of the programs that we have developed. Our programs for teaching imitation and meaning are two of the most basic kinds of procedures employed in the course of an extensive effort at helping these children to use language. The programs for imitation and meaning have been used with almost every child we have seen. However, many of the children have been taught behaviors as complex as verb transformations (changing verbs from present to past tense), pluralization, sentence formation, conversational speech, storytelling, and a score of other intellectual and social skills. A complete review of our efforts in the area of language acquisition may be found on film (Lovaas, 1969) and in a forthcoming text (Lovaas, 1974).

TEACHING LANGUAGE SKILLS

With most children, the problem of teaching speech never arises—speech develops without anyone knowing much about how it happens. It is a "natural" phenomenon, and knowledge of the process is, for practical reasons, usually not necessary. Unfortunately some children do not learn to talk on their own. They need help, and we are left in a disappointing position because we do not know how language is acquired. People have, however, made guesses about what transpires, and one of these guesses is that experience is central in producing language; that is, that language is learned. We made a concerted attempt to show that language can be created in a nonspeaking person through the manipulation of environmental events. We outline here a procedure by which speech can be taught to previously mute children. Undoubtedly, there are, or will be, other ways to accomplish the same goal, however; the program we detail includes two basic phases: (a) the establishment of vocal behaviors in previously mute children (verbal imitation), and (b) the establishment of an appropriate context for speech (meaning).

Before we begin to describe the specific procedures that we employ, the reader should become familiar with some of the technical terms. We define terms and outline procedures in some detail to illustrate the highly organized, rather meticulous manner in which we set about teaching children. Readers familiar with laboratory research on learning will realize just how extensively we have relied upon such research in designing our program.

The term *training stimulus* will be used frequently. A training stimulus is a stimulus to which one teaches a correct response. Such a training stimulus may be nonverbal (such as an object like a cup, or a behavior—like jumping), or it may be verbal (e.g., a question or a command), or it may be, and usually is, a combination of verbal and nonverbal elements. For example, an attending adult may present an object (such as a cup) and ask a question (e.g., "What is this?").

Prompts and *prompt fading* are crucial elements in our procedures. A prompt is a stimulus that cues the desired response prior to training, or with minimal training. A prompt facilitates the child's response in the presence of the training stimulus so that one can begin reinforcement. Without prompts, the child may never give the desired response. When one presents a prompt, one becomes a participant in the child's response in some sense. Prompting may be accomplished in a variety of ways. The teacher may physically direct the child to perform some response, or may tell the child the correct answer. At other times, the teacher may serve as a model for the child's behavior. For example, if the desired response is nonverbal, like touching an object, the teacher may prompt the desired response by picking up the child's hand and placing it on the correct object. If the child is imitating reliably, the teacher might prompt the desired response by touching the object himself and then reinforcing the child for imitation. If the response is verbal, the teacher might make the desired response himself, and reinforce the child for imitation.

After the response has been prompted for several trials, the prompt is slowly eliminated, and the training stimulus remains. This process of elimination is called fading the prompt, and, as the term implies, it is a gradual process in most cases. Over a number of trials, the teacher decreases his participation in the child's response. For example, in the case of a nonverbal prompt, such as moving the child's hand toward the object, the teacher might move the child's hand only three-fourths of the way toward the object, then one-half the way, then simply touch the child's hand. If the prompt is verbal, the teacher might gradually lower the decibel level of the prompt, then give only the initial sound, and then voicelessly form the initial sound with the lips. After a number of trials, the teacher discontinues presenting the prompt entirely.

A *correct response* may be said to occur when the child is making the desired response to the training stimulus without prompts. The reader should note that we cannot say with any confidence that the child is responding "to the training stimulus" merely because he emitted the desired response at the appropriate time. The child could be responding to some aspect of the teacher's behavior such as the tone of the teacher's voice or the way the teacher looks at the training stimulus. Until a discrimination has been made, that is, until the child is giving the desired response to one training stimulus and not to another, we have no reason to believe he is responding to the training stimulus. We attempt to accomplish this discrimination in the next phase of the procedure.

Stimulus rotation describes the way in which the second training stimulus is introduced and presented. After the child begins responding "reliably" to the first training stimulus (TS1), the child is meeting some criterion level of performance, such as 10 consecutive desired responses without a prompt. Let us say that TS1 is the command, "Raise your arm." When the child is raising his arm reliably upon command, the teacher introduces a second command, such as, "Stand up." The child will almost certainly give the first response R1 (raise his arm), when the new command is first presented. The teacher corrects the child, prompts the new desired response, fades the prompt, and drills the child to criterion on the new command.

When the child has mastered the response to the second training stimulus, the teacher now presents the first training stimulus TS1 ("Raise your arm") again. Now the child will usually give R2 (stand up). The teacher again corrects the child and drills to criterion. One finds that the number of errors the child makes in switching from TS1 to TS2 decreases each time the teacher changes the training stimulus. When the child makes no more than one incorrect response after the teacher switches the training stimuli, the teacher proceeds to nonsystematic rotation. The means that the teacher presents TS1 and TS2 in an unpredictable order. Once the child is able to respond to the training stimuli correctly when they are presented in nonsystematic order, one can say that the child is making a "correct response" and proceed to introduce TS3, TS4, and so on.

VERBAL IMITATION

Let us now turn to a more specific description of our method for teaching the child verbal behavior. In our earliest work, we had attempted to teach the children to emit sounds and words through the direct shaping of vocalizations. This means that we reinforced random vocalizations, raising the frequency of their occurrence, and subsequently reinforced only those sounds that were more and more similar to the sounds we had preselected. This procedure is similar to that used by Hayes (1951) to establish a three-word vocabulary in a chimpanzee, and to that employed by Isaacs, Thomas, and Golddiamond (1960) as well as Sherman (1965) in *reinstating* verbal behavior in adult schizophrenics. Although the children we worked with learned a few words in this manner, it became clear that, despite extensive efforts, they could acquire only a limited vocabulary if we continued to use such a procedure.

Casual observation suggests the possibility that normal children learn much of their speech through the imitation of the speech that they hear adults use, rather than through direct shaping. Mute autistic children do not imitate; therefore, it seemed a potentially practical starting point to attempt to teach these children to imitate. The method we eventually found most efficient can be described as a discrimination learning procedure. It can be said that discrimination learning obtains when a behavior occurs in the presence of certain features of a stimulus and not in their absence. It should be clear now that we have defined "correct response" for the purpose of our program as a "discriminated response."

Although Baer and Sherman (1964) were primarily interested in imitation in normal children, their conceptualization of the acquisition of imitation in terms of reinforcement theory helped us to establish a framework for teaching imitation to nonimitating children. Briefly, Baer and Sherman viewed the acquisition of imitation as the acquisition of a discrimination in which the topological similarity between an adult's behavior and a child's behavior becomes the discriminative stimulus for reinforcement. The child must learn to attend to the correspondence between his actions and the adult's actions. Accordingly, we set out to bring the child's vocalizations under the control of the adult's vocalizations and ultimately to teach the child that similarity between his vocalizations and those of the adult was the discriminative stimulus for reinforcement.

We approached this task in four distinct phases. Before one can gain control of a behavior, that behavior must occur with reasonable frequency. Therefore, in the first phase, the child was reinforced for all vocalizations. During this phase, the child was also reinforced for visually fixating on the adult's mouth.

Phase 2 included the initial attempts that we made to bring the child's vocalizations under the control of the adult's. The child was first required to learn a temporal discrimination. He was reinforced if and only if he vocalized within six seconds after the adult's vocalization.

In the third phase, we began to require that the child's vocalizations match those of the adult. The child was reinforced for only those sounds which were increasingly similar to the adult's. To carry out successfully this phase of the procedure, we found it necessary to select sounds that could be prompted. One can open a child's mouth, hold down his tongue, and thus prompt him to produce the sound "ah," or some reasonable facsimile. One can then hold the child's mouth closed and prompt him to produce the sound "mm." These two sounds are not only easily prompted, but also they are appropriate as initial training stimuli because they have distinctive visual cues when produced by another person. We found that sounds like "k," and "g," without these features, were far more difficult to teach.

Once the initial sounds were selected, teaching followed closely the basic pattern of stimulus presentation which was described as *stimulus rotation*. The teacher waits for the child to look at the teacher's mouth, and then presents TS1 (in this case the sound "ah"). The desired response is prompted, and the prompt is faded over subsequent trials. TS1 is presented repeatedly until the child reaches criterion. The teacher then introduces TS2 ("mm"), prompts the desired response, fades the prompt, and so on. The teacher returns to TS1, regains the first response ("ah"), presents TS2 again, and so on. Once the child can match these two sounds when they are presented in nonsystematic order, the teacher begins to train new sounds and words. Procedures for adding new training stimuli will vary depending on the child. Sometimes, the teacher may simply present a new sound in nonsystematic order with previously acquired sounds, and the child will quickly master the new material. With other children, the teacher may have to repeat the procedure from the first step: training new sounds singly, then systematically rotating them with one or two old sounds, and finally proceding to nonsystematic rotation. Even when the child imme- diately imitates a new sound, it is usually necessary to rehearse previously mas- tered material from time to time. Previously mastered sounds and words are re- hearsed in nonsystematic order on a schedule which suits the individual child. Usually, one previously mastered sound every five to six trials is adequate. However, some children require more extensive review.

We have exposed all of the mute children we have seen to this imitation training program in one- to two-hour sessions once or twice a day. These chil- dren varied enormously in the rate with which they acquired imitative vocal be- havior, but all of them learned something. The learning curve for every child showed positive acceleration and savings over tasks; that is, all of the children appeared to "learn to learn." Some children acquired elaborate imitative behav- ior in one or two weeks. Others required extensive training. Billy and Chuck are two of the most profoundly disturbed children we have seen, yet in some regards, their performance was typical. The data for the first 26 days of imita- tion training for these two children are plotted in Figure 1. The abscissa denotes days of training. The words and sounds are printed in lower case letters on the days when they were introduced and practiced and in capital letters on the day they were mastered, that is, on the day when the child reached criterion. One can clearly see that the rate of mastery increased as the training progressed. While it took several days to train a single word in the first two weeks of the program, several words were learned on each day of the last two weeks. The positive acceleration of this curve is typical of the form of acquisition curves for all of the children.

Another interesting kind of data that we obtained on the acquisition of verbal imitation concern, the nature of the errors the children made. Figure 2 presents the errors occuring in successive imitative responses for a five-year-old initially mute boy, Jose. The figure shows disruption in the performance of previously acquired imitation with the introduction of new sounds. Consider the disruption of "ah" in Session 2, where the second sound, "mm," was introduced. The performance of "ah" was also disrupted when the third sound, "eh," was in- troduced (Session 16). The same phenomena occurred in Session 24 when the fourth sound, "agogoha," was presented. Similar effects can be observed in "mm" when "eh" was introduced, and so on. The disruption in previously mastered sounds was less severe with each new training stimulus. Some very similar data for meaning training are presented later. The similarities between errors that occur in these two programs suggest that the same process is operat- ing in both kinds of acquisition. This process is discrimination learning.

When the child completed imitation training, he was able to produce the verbalizations which he heard, but the productions were without meaning be- cause they did not have a context. The word "mama" has no meaning for a

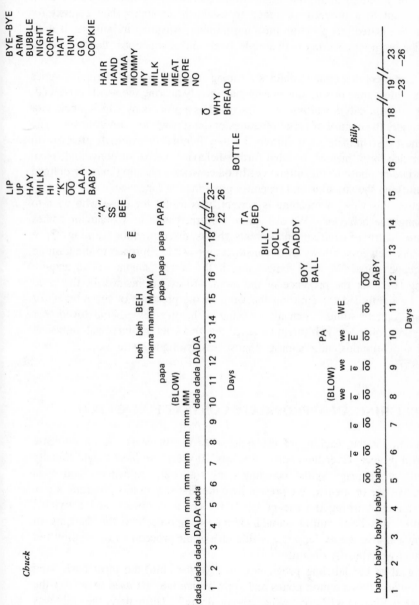

Figure 1. The first 26 days of verbal imitation for two previously mute children. Sounds and words appear in lower case on the days they were introduced and practiced, and in upper case on the day when they were mastered. From O. I. Lovaas et al., Acquisition of imitative speech by schizophrenic children, *Science*, February 11, 1966, **151**, 705–707, Fig. 1. Copyright 1966 by the American Association for the Advancement of Science.

181

child if he only echos it and never emits it or responds to it (for instance by smiling or pointing) in any other situation. Therefore, we introduced the child at this point to a program designed to establish an appropriate context for speech. We called this program meaning training. Meaning training itself is an extensive program covering both simple labels and abstractions, that is, semantics.

The argument that context defines meaning suggests that the utterance comes under a wider range of stimulus events than merely hearing the words produced. Earlier, discrimination learning was described as a process by which a behavior comes under the control of certain features of the surrounding environment. The child must discriminate what stimuli, be they internal or external, give rise to an utterance like "mama" or what further behavior, verbal or nonverbal, is an appropriate response to this utterance. In other words, meaning may be defined by identifying the stimulus and response properties of language.

Whether this view of meaning is correct, it is useful for those who wish to build language behaviors. We are again concerned with how behavior comes under the control of environmental events, that is, discrimination learning. Once again, this viewpoint allows us to construct a plausible approach to the training of language skills. We may expect that if the word "mama" is to acquire meaning (i.e., for the presence of the mother to evoke this word), the child should be reinforced for emitting the word in the presence of the mother (or other appropriate stimuli such as a feeling of helplessness, being loved, her coming and going, etc.). It might be noted that this kind of functional-empirical definition of stimulus and response is most closely aligned with Skinner's position (1957).

ESTABLISHING AN APPROPRIATE CONTEXT FOR SPEECH

A program for the teaching of the appropriate use of speech is an immense long-term project. Over the course of nearly 10 years, we have taught literally hundreds of language skills including conversational, expository, and even imaginative use of speech. We present here the first step in this program: a procedure for establishing the use of labels for common objects and activities. Hopefully, this brief outline should clarify our approach to the teaching of meaning and give the reader a reasonable idea of the procedures we employ and the results we typically obtain.

The goal of the labeling program is to give the child the most basic kind of vocabulary: the common nouns and verbs which may be used to answer the questions, "What is it?" and "What are you doing?" Ultimately, the child was taught to give verbal answers to these questions, however, as in many of the procedures that we developed, we found it advantageous to first train the child

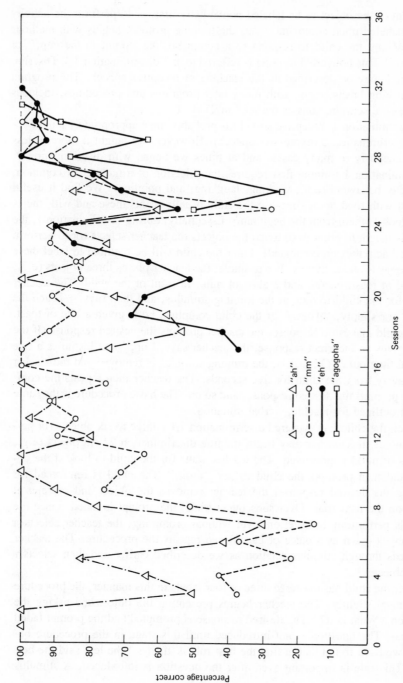

Figure 2. The acquisition of four initial sounds in a previously mute child. Number of sessions appears on the abscissa. Sessions occurred twice a day and lasted about one hour. Percentage of correct, unprompted responses appears on the ordinate.

to identify the object to be labeled nonverbally first, or to perform the activity to be labeled upon command. Thus the training protocol begins with methods for teaching the child to respond to a command like "point to the cup," or "jump." This nonverbal training is referred to as "discrimination 1." Discrimination 1 may be described as the teaching of receptive speech. The program for teaching labels, along with many later programs and procedures, includes two basic discriminations as outlined in Table 1.

Discrimination 1 (receptive speech) is probably most appropriately taught before discrimination 2 (expressive speech). However, we taught it more or less simultaneously in many cases, and at times we began with discrimination 2. Discrimination 1 training first requires the selection of a number of common, everyday behaviors (e.g., walking, laughing, and pointing). We find it useful to start with food items, because the child usually wants these and will, therefore, look at them from the beginning. Essentially, during discrimination 1, the child is taught to point to or touch the objects the teacher selects (or to perform selected activities on command). Later the child will be required to label these same objects and activities. For example, the teacher places three objects (e.g., a piece of toast, bacon, and a glass of milk) in front of the child. The teacher waits for the child to look at the training stimulus, and then says, "Touch the toast," or simply, "Toast." If the child complies, he is given a bite of toast. If the child makes no response, the teacher prompts the desired response. If the child gives an incorrect response, the teacher says, "no," and institutes a five second time out (TO); that is, the training stimulus is removed and the teacher turns away from the child for five seconds. The teacher then repeats the command, prompts the desired response, and so on. The basic procedure is the same as that outlined for teaching verbal imitation.

When the child has mastered discrimination 1 for three to six objects (or perhaps more), the teacher may begin training discrimination 2. An object (e.g., a glass of milk) is presented. The teacher waits for the child to look at the object, and then prompts the child to say "milk." The child is reinforced for making the desired response, the teacher removes the object and presents it again on the next trial. Over subsequent trials, the prompt is faded. Once the child is performing at criterion level without prompting, the teacher selects a new object (such as a piece of bacon) and repeats the procedure. The teacher proceeds through stimulus rotation as we described earlier and then selects a third object.

After the child has mastered three or four labels in this manner, the procedure is changed slightly. The teacher begins presenting the object and asking the question "What is it?" The desired response is prompted and the prompt faded as usual. The question is not introduced until this stage in the procedure because we have found that at first the best rule is always "the less said the better." This rule is important even after the question is introduced. A stimulus

Table 1.   Outline of the Language Training Program

Discrimination	Stimulus	Response	Examples
1. (receptive speech)	Verbal behavior of self or others	Nonverbal	Instructions (giving or receiving)
2. (expressive speech)	Nonverbal Objects Symbols Behavior of self or others	Verbal	Labeling, or describing environment Testing Describing behavior of self or others

such as "What is this John, look at me, hey, look over here, what is this?" has probably lost, or perhaps never acquired, any stimulus functions.

When the child has mastered a small labeling vocabulary, perhaps a dozen words or so, generalization training begins. The child is exposed to numerous examples of a class of objects that he has learned to label (e.g., many chairs). In this way, he learns that chairs come in many colors and shapes and materials. One can argue that the child has a "concept" when he can label instances of a class of objects the first time they are presented.

Of course, it is impossible to bring hundreds of chairs into the laboratory for the purpose of generalization training, but the outside world contains chairs in more than sufficient number, so it becomes efficient to make teaching the child part of his everyday life. At some point this transfer of training from the laboratory to everyday life occurs in every program that we teach. Language is too rich to be taught exclusively in the lab, but we find it necessary to begin with the controlled procedures of the lab to better assess what difficulties the child has and thereby to be in a better position to remediate.

At this point, data illustrating the results we typically obtain in teaching a child to label may be illustrative. The acquisition of simple labels by two of the children who were initially mute, Kevin (age seven) and Taylor (age five), is presented in Figure 3. These children received several months of training in verbal imitation before labels were taught. Labels are presented in the figure in lower case letters on the days when they were introduced and practiced, and in capital case when they were mastered. As in Figure 1, it took several days for the children to learn a particular label in the beginning, yet they acquired several labels in a single day later on in training. Again, one sees the positive acceleration of the learning curves ("learning to learn"), the same acceleration evident in Figure 1 and in data for all the children we have taught.

As the program continued, many of the children eventually acquired new labels on the basis of a single trial. To put it another way, once the child was told what response was desired, he would then answer correctly on all subsequent trials. Yet it must be noted that the shape of the curves varied enormously between children. For example, Taylor (Figure 3) might require 40 days to

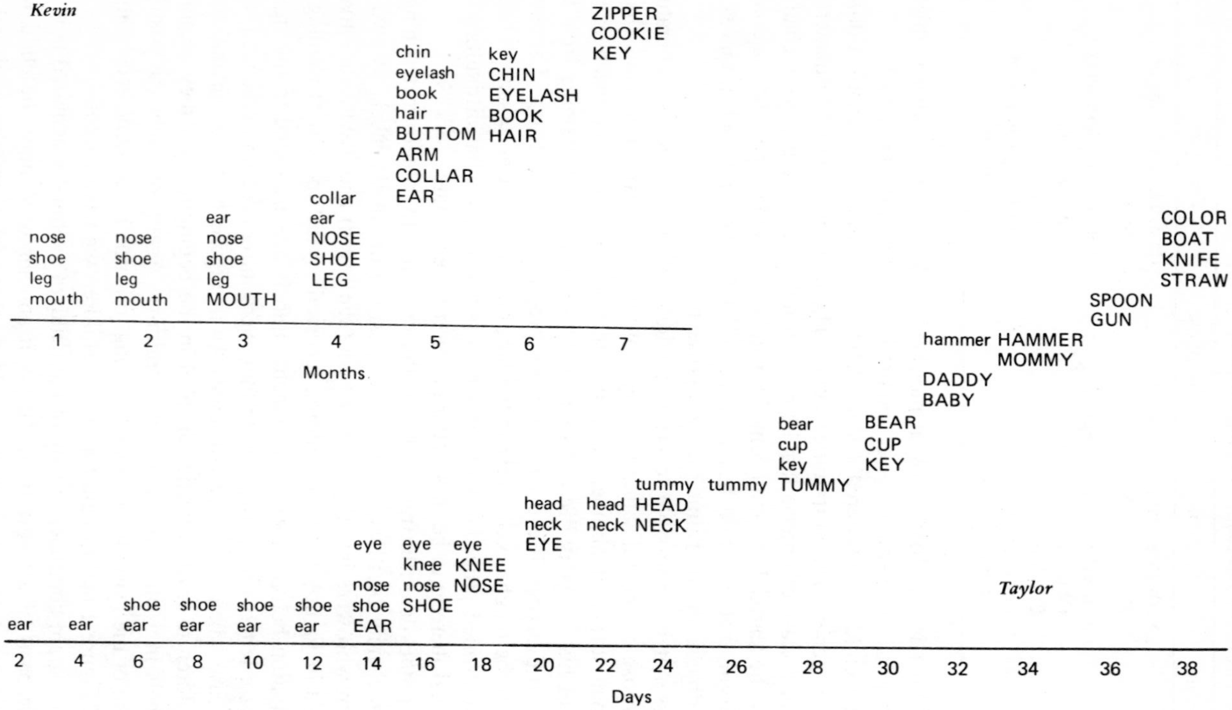

Kevin

ZIPPER
COOKIE
KEY

	chin	key
	eyelash	CHIN
	book	EYELASH
	hair	BOOK
	BUTTOM	HAIR
	ARM	
	COLLAR	
	EAR	

nose	nose	ear	collar		
shoe	shoe	nose	ear		
leg	leg	shoe	NOSE		
mouth	mouth	leg	SHOE		
		MOUTH	LEG		

| 1 | 2 | 3 | 4 | 5 | 6 | 7 |

Months

COLOR
BOAT
KNIFE
STRAW

SPOON
GUN

hammer HAMMER
        MOMMY

        DADDY
        BABY

bear BEAR
cup CUP
key KEY
TUMMY

tummy HEAD
head NECK
neck

head eye eye
neck eye KNEE
EYE knee nose NOSE
    nose shoe SHOE
    shoe EAR
    ear

| ear | ear | shoe | shoe | shoe | shoe | eye | | | | | | | | | | | | |
| ear | | ear | ear | ear | ear | nose | | | | | | | | | | | | |

| 2 | 4 | 6 | 8 | 10 | 12 | 14 | 16 | 18 | 20 | 22 | 24 | 26 | 28 | 30 | 32 | 34 | 36 | 38 |

Days

Taylor

Figure 3. The acquisition of labels by two previously mute children. Labels appear in lower case on the days when they were introduced and practiced, in upper case on the day when they were mastered.

186

master the same material an echolalic child could master within one or two days. In fact, in the early stages of this program, prior to more objective data collection, we taught the alphabet (26 paired associates) to an eight-year-old echolalic child in less than two hours. A performance like that, which may be matched by a typical college freshman, can sometimes be observed among autistics. Often, however, it may take a year to teach that much using our current procedures.

A child may make very slow progress for a variety of reasons. Part of the problem may be attributable to imprecise application of the procedures described here; part of the problem lies in the nature of the procedure itself. To use the procedure correctly, one must constantly be watching for any one of a number of wrong responses the child may learn. If the teacher provides extra cues—a smile, a nod, a word—the child may learn to respond to these rather than the training stimulus. The child may learn to alternate his responses—that is, if his first response is not reinforced, he immediately makes a different response—continuing to run through his repertoire until some response is reinforced. If a verbal response is being taught, the child may produce unintelligible sounds or become inaudible if the teacher reinforces near approximations. Great care is necessary to insure that the child is responding to the training stimulus and that the response is clear, discrete, and correct.

In the beginning, we quickly discovered exactly how difficult it can be to teach even a seemingly simple discrimination properly. For example, in one case a child required 90,000 trials to label bacon and milk correctly. This does not imply that operant conditioning is necessarily a slow process, but rather, may well illustrate the teacher's ignorance of how to teach efficiently. The child in this instance learned to change to a different response when his first response was not reinforced. In other words, his self-correction was controlled by whether his first response was reinforced, rather than by the nature of the training stimulus. He became dependent upon the prompt; that is, he would not respond unless prompted and would "search" for the most subtle of visual cues from the teacher. Some children perseverate; others become barely audible. Wasserman (1969) has described some of the problems that autistic children exhibit during discrimination training.

These problems are partially responsible for a series of studies from our lab in the last few years which deal with a phenomenon we have labeled stimulus overselectivity (Lovaas, Schreibman, Koegel, & Rehm, 1971; Lovaas & Schreibman, 1971; Koegal & Whilhelm, 1971; Koegal, 1971; Schreibman & Lovaas, 1973). Stimulus overselectivity refers to the fact that, when presented with a complex stimulus in a discrimination task, autistic children typically respond on the basis of only one of the components of the stimulus. This finding has some important implications for designing optimal teaching programs for autistic children. It suggests that the provision of certain kinds of prompts may not facilitate discrimination learning in autistics.

Recent evidence on prompting and overselectivity (Schreibman, 1972) demonstrates quite clearly that while autistic children do not acquire discriminations without prompting, certain types of prompts are very much better than others. The reader will notice that in the examples presented so far, the prompts described were stimuli which the teacher presents *in addition* to the training stimulus. Schreibman refers to these prompts as "extra-stimulus" prompts. In contrast, a within-stimulus prompt is accomplished by simply emphasizing the relevant feature of the training stimulus itself.

It may be helpful to present an example of the use of a within-stimulus prompt. If the discrimination to be taught is between the words "tall" and "ball," one might prompt the desired response by pointing to the word simultaneous with the verbal production of the word. Such a procedure uses an extra-stimulus prompt. Alternatively, one might begin by presenting the letter T, in large, bold print, slowly fade in a large, bold **B**, then proceed to fade in the remaining three letters, and finally reduce the emphases on the two initial letters. This alternative procedure illustrates the use of within-stimulus prompt; the critical component of the discrimination itself is emphasized, and then this emphasis is faded.

Schreibman's study supports our earlier casual observations that autistic children often become too dependent on certain prompts. The children in her study often exhibited difficulty when required to produce the correct response to the training stimulus alone after complete fading of the extra-stimulus prompt. This inability to shift control of behavior from one aspect of the environment to another is the basic finding of research on overselectivity. Autistic children appear to be unable to attend to multiple cues simultaneously. If an extra-stimulus prompt is to facilitate learning, a child must, in fact, attend to more than one cue. The within-stimulus prompt does not require the child to respond to multiple cues, and is, therefore, a greatly superior facilitator of learning for autistic children. As we develop within-stimulus prompts, we expect to increase substantially the efficiency of the programs and procedures outlined in this chapter.

Over the years, we have taught a vast number of behaviors involving the child's discriminations of relatively simple stimulus aspects of the environment. In each case, the acquisition was positively accelerated. Consider the acquisition of correct responses to simple commands, such as "raise arm," "touch belly," "clap hands," "stand up," "touch nose," "tongue out," "touch eye," "touch ear," and "pat head." For Michael (a six-year-old mute autistic), the number of sessions required for acquisition were 4, 3, 2, 2, 3, 1, 2, 1, 1, and 1, respectively. For correct responses to simple questions: "What do you want?" ("Cookie"); "What's your name?" ("Mike"); "What is this?" ("Baby"); "How are you?" ("Fine"); "Do you want [name of a food]?"

("Yes"); "Do you want me to hit you?" ("No"), the number of sessions Michael required was 9, 8, 3, 4, 4, and 3, respectively. The absolute number of sessions differs between children, but the data for Michael are representative of the data for mute children, and the accelerated rate of acquisition is characteristic of the data for all children.

The errors that the child makes as new stimuli are introduced give some clue to the underlying learning process. We collected data on the deterioration of performance for one label when a new label was introduced for Michael and Jose. These data are presented in Figure 4. Both Mike and Jose were initially mute and both were approximately five years old at the time these data were collected. The ordinate shows percentage correct responses, and the number of sessions are shown on the abscissa. Sessions took place twice a day, one in the morning and one in the afternoon. Figure 4 makes it quite clear that whenever a new label was introduced, it interfered with the production of one introduced previously, and that new labels produced less interference as the number of labels mastered increased. The similarity to the results described in Figure 2 (errors during the acquisition of verbal imitation) suggests that both of these acquisitions are broadly based on discrimination learning, rather than examples of some narrower category like "language learning," or some limiting feature of the material.

Returning to Figure 4, consider the fact that the first label was learned quickly, and immediately became the most likely response to any and all objects which were presented to the child. The difficulties began when we attempted to establish a discriminated response; for example, when the second label was introduced. Once the child was able to discriminate verbally between the first two objects, subsequent discriminations proceeded with more ease, until the child sometimes reached the stage where the teacher had only to label an object once before the child learned. It appears that the child learns to discriminate which aspects of the environment are associated with labels, and to respond only to those features which define objects. Clearly, to focus or guide the attention of the child in this way requires considerable differential reinforcement.

Labeling is a continuous process. The larger the child's vocabulary, the more flexible the teacher can be in introducing new tasks and teaching new labels. Once the child acquires a basic labeling vocabulary, composed primarily of nouns and verbs, he may be taught to respond to more abstract stimuli. We teach the children to respond to pronouns, prepositions, color labels, words for size, shape, and quantity (more, less), words for temporal relationships (first, last, before, after), the use of yes and no, and such. The basic procedures involved in these programs are essentially the same as those outlined for labeling. The teacher presents a training stimulus, prompts the desired response, fades the prompt, introduces a new stimulus, and so on. For example, in teaching prepositions, the teacher presents the child with a penny in a cup and asks the ques-

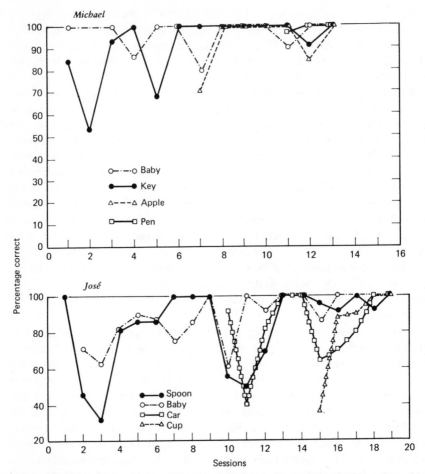

Figure 4. The acquisition of the first four labels for two critically mute children. The number of sessions appears on the abscissa. Sessions occurred twice a day and lasted about one hour. The percentage of correct, unprompted responses appears on the ordinate.

tion "Where is the penny?" The answer, "In the cup," is prompted, and so on. The data that we have obtained on the acquisition of simple abstractions reflect the same positive acceleration and savings over tasks that was characteristic of data on both imitation and labeling.

The major difference between the procedures for labeling and those for teaching abstractions lies in the nature of the training stimulus. In teaching abstractions, the training stimuli are often very much more complex than those used for teaching common labels. The training stimuli for abstractions may be differences in the number of objects in various groups (e.g., a larger pile of objects and a small pile used to teach "more" and "less"), a spatial relationship between objects (a penny "in" a cup), or the relationship between two events occurring at different points in time (e.g., the teacher instructs the child to touch the boat and then to touch the car).

Training in imitation, labeling, or any program rarely proceeds smoothly. Despite the problems, however, we can teach some of the basic skills involved in linguistic behavior to nonlinguistic children using the principles of learning theory. Over the past 10 years, we have presented data illustrating the acquisition of many specific linguistic skills, and have also attempted to assess the results of the total program provided for the children. We developed a method of measurement designed to provide general information about changes in both verbal and nonverbal behavior during treatment. This method of measurement allows the assessment of generalization across situations and behaviors as well as over time (follow-up). Our attempt at assessment is a long-term effort, and the data often span the entire period the project has been in operation.

GENERALIZATION AND FOLLOW-UP MEASURES

Baer, Wolf, and Risley (1968) present a position similar to the one we adopted in designing a measure of treatment effects. Such a framework dictates that measurement of changes during treatment should include three areas of assessment: (1) measures of stimulus generalization, or the extent to which behavior changes that occur in the treatment environment transfer to situations outside that environment; (2) response generalization, or the extent to which changes in a limited set of behaviors effect changes in a larger range of behaviors; and (3) generalizations over time (durability) or how well therapeutic effects are maintained over time.

The reader will find a comprehensive discussion of our viewpoint, the data, and the relevant literature in Lovaas, Koegal, Simmons, and Stevens-Long (1973). We here present a brief outline of this effort. By now, the reader should have an idea of the major interventions that we attempted. In general, we sought to extinguish or suppress pathological behaviors and to teach socially desirable behaviors. We tried to decrease the frequency of self-destructive and self-stimulatory behavior as well as tantrums and similar disruptive acts. We hoped to teach appropriate verbal behavior. At the same time we attempted to teach speech, we also began programs designed to help the child learn social and self-help behaviors, from showing affection to table manners, brushing the teeth and playing games (Lovaas, 1967). In short, we tried to teach these children what middle-class parents of the western world try to teach theirs.

To gain perspective on the data and the potential of the system of measurement that we developed, one should be familiar with some of the general limitations encountered while assessing therapeutic effects with autistic children in our specific treatment environment. Our program was developed primarily as a research program, not primarily as a treatment center. We have heavily emphasized language training, even though this may not have resulted in maximal positive gains in therapy. We have often withheld aspects of treatment to more reliably assess their potential effectiveness. We usually selected the children with the poorest prognosis. Finally, we never developed liason with facilities in the community which might have provided foster home placement or special schooling for the children we treated once they were discharged. With these reservations in mind, we present a summary of our measures of treatment effectiveness.

We have used two kinds of measures: a multiple response recording and changes in test scores on the children's Stanford-Binet and Vineland Social Maturity Scale. The main focus of our assessment efforts has been on the multiple response recordings which primarily provide information on stimulus generalization and the duration of treatment effects. The test scores provide more general information on both stimulus and response generalization.

Multiple-Response Recordings

The basic procedure for this measure involves defining certain behaviors (both normal and pathological) for an observer *(O)* who then records their frequency and duration. In our lab, recording was done on a button panel coupled to a computer tape punch.

The psychotic children we have treated display limited behavioral repertoires; therefore, the problem of defining and reliably categorizing their behavior is somewhat simplified. We eventually decided upon five behavioral categories which seem optimally useful in describing autistic children. (1) *Self-stimulation.* This is stereotyped, repetitive behavior that appears only to provide the child with proprioceptive feedback, including such behaviors as flapping the arms, rocking, spinning, twirling objects, crossing or rolling the eyes, gazing and grimacing, and so on. (2) *Echolalic speech.* This occurs when a child echos the speech of others, either immediately or after a delay, giving the impression of nonrelated, inappropriate speech. Such speech is often characterized by pronoun reversal, incorrect use of tense, and such. This category was also used to record instances of bizarre words and word combinations. (3) *Appropriate speech.* This is understandable, grammatically correct speech, related to an appropriate context. (4) *Social nonverbal behavior.* This refers to appropriate nonverbal behavior that is dependent upon cues given by another person for its initiation or completion (e.g., responding to requests or imitating). (5) *Appropriate play.* This is defined as the use of toys and objects in an appropriate, age-related manner.

The *O*s were given very detailed definitions of each of these behaviors and numerous examples were provided. They were told that if they were unsure about whether an observed behavior fit into a particular category, they should not record anything. The *O*s were instructed to press a button on the button panel which was labeled with the category of behavior they were observing and hold down the button until the child terminated that behavior.

To assess stimulus generalization, the children were observed in a room separate from our training facilities and in the company of an unfamiliar adult. A number of toys were present in the room (a wagon, paper and crayons, a bobo doll, a large rubber ball, etc.). The children were observed for a total of 35 minutes. During the first 10 minutes, the child was observed while alone in the room (this condition will be referred to as "alone"). During the second 10 minutes ("attending"), an unfamiliar adult was present in the room and attended to the child visually, but initiated no interaction, made no comments, and interfered in no way unless the child initiated some activity requiring interaction with the adult. If the child initiated such activity, the adult performed those responses necessary to complete the interaction. In the final 15 minutes ("inviting"), the adult encouraged the child to engage in a variety of activities. The adult invited the child to play in turn with each of 11 toys, demonstrating for one minute the use of each toy. The adult attempted to initiate a game of "pattycake," gave the child a one-minute series of simple commands which could be performed nonverbally (e.g., "sit down"), and then asked the child a one-minute series of questions requiring purely verbal answers (e.g., "What's your name?").

A summary of changes during treatment for all of the children is presented in Figure 5. Before *(B)* and after *(A)* multiple response measures are averaged over all conditions for the total group, as well as for mute and echolalic children separately. Percentage occurrence of each category of behavior is plotted on the ordinate. Behavioral categories are given on the abscissa. *E* refers to the average results for the echolalic children, *M* to the average results for the mute children, and *T* to the average results for the total group.

Figure 5 clearly indicates that, when before and after measures are compared, inappropriate behaviors decrease while appropriate behaviors increase. Self-stimulation decreased by about two-thirds for the group as a whole. As a group, the children showed about four times as much appropriate play and three times as much appropriate social nonverbal behavior as they exhibited before treatment. It should be underlined that there were no exceptions. All the children improved.

For the purposes of reporting the results of these measurement sessions, the children are best considered in four groups: in Group 1, Ricky, Pam, Billy, and Chuck, were observed "before" treatment (June 1964) and then on a monthly schedule during 14 subsequent months of treatment. All four children were hospitalized within one year after discharge from our program in the same state hospital. Pam and Ricky were returned for follow-up in 1968 and given a brief period of treatment at that time. They were then discharged again to the state hospital. They returned once more for observation in 1970. Chuck and Billy were observed after discharge once, in 1970.

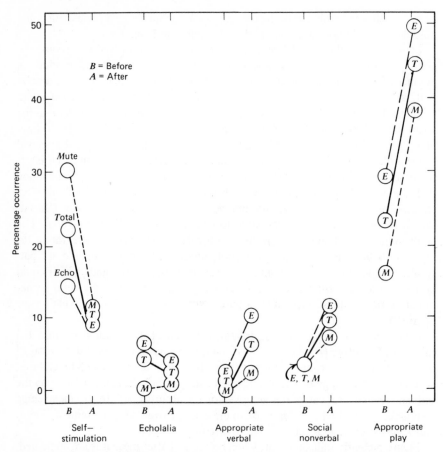

Figure 5. Percentage occurrence of multiple response measure behavioral categories for echolalic children *(E)*, mute children *(M)*, and the two groups combined *(I)*, before *(B)* and after *(A)* treatment. From O. I. Lovaas, R. Koegal, J. Q. Simons, and J. Stevens-Long, Some generalization and followup measures on autistic children in behavior therapy, *Journal of Applied Behavior Analysis*, 1973, **6**, 131–166, Fig. 1. Copyright 1973 by the Society for the Experimental Analysis of Behavior, Inc.

Three children fall in Group 2 (Jose, Michael, and Taylor). They were observed before treatment (1966) and every three months thereafter during a 12-month treatment program. They returned for follow-up measures in 1970.

The third and fourth groups were seen as outpatients. Seth, Leslie, and Tito (Group 3) were observed before treatment (1968), after one year of treatment, and then received follow-up measures in 1970. The fourth group (Kevin F., Ann, and James) were observed before treatment (1969) and after one year (1970).

One of the major differences in the treatment programs between groups is the degree of training that we gave the parents in the role of therapist. Parents began to serve as therapists in Group 2, although the involvement of Group 2 parents was minimal (the children were in-patients). Parents of the third and fourth groups were trained in shaping procedures in the clinic, and then we served primarily as consultants to the parents. They became the primary therapists for their own child.

We assessed the rate of change during treatment by analyzing the monthly measures collected for Group 1. The data show, for example, that spontaneous initiation of social interaction and verbal contact (which can be assessed most easily by examining the data for the ''attending'' condition) occurred after about eight months of treatment. Results also indicated that the children show more social nonverbal behavior than language behavior and only two children (Ricky and Billy) engaged in spontaneous verbal behavior in the attending condition.

Group 2 children differ from the other groups in some important ways. First, all of the children in Group 2 was initially mute. Moreover, although the children in Group 2 were in-patients, the treatment program for these children differed from Group 1 in that the first six months of the Group 2 program was less intensive. We tried to use no aversive stimulation and to use a less demanding schedule. After six months, we returned to the more demanding schedule because the children made little definite progress in the first six months. The results for Group 2 were essentially the same as those for Group 1, except that Group 2 showed only minimal improvement in verbal behavior.

The data for Groups 3 and 4 reflected the same decreases in inappropriate behaviors and increases in appropriate ones consistent with the data for Groups 1 and 2.

Turning to the follow-up data, comparisons between groups become especially instructive. Since the parents of the children in Groups 2, 3, and 4 were trained in the use of shaping techniques, this group of parents were prepared, in varying degrees, to extend the child's program beyond the limited experience we could offer. Figure 6 presents multiple response follow-up measures for Group 1 children, as well as for the parent-trained groups. Percentage occurrence of the various categories of behavior is plotted on the ordinate for Before (B) and After (A) treatment, and for most recent follow-up (F) measures. I refers to the average result for the four children in Group 1, and P refers to the average result for the six children in Groups 2 and 3 (follow-up data for Group 4 is not available yet). For all categories of appropriate behavior, the data indicate that the children in Group 1 lost what they had gained in treatment. Figure 6 shows social nonverbal behavior, appropriate verbal behavior, and appropriate play behavior decreased, while psychotic behavior increased. Children whose parents had been trained maintained gains made during treatment, and some of these children continued to improve after discharge.

As was mentioned earlier, Ricky and Pam were observed again in 1968. At that time, we decided to return them to intensive treatment for a short period

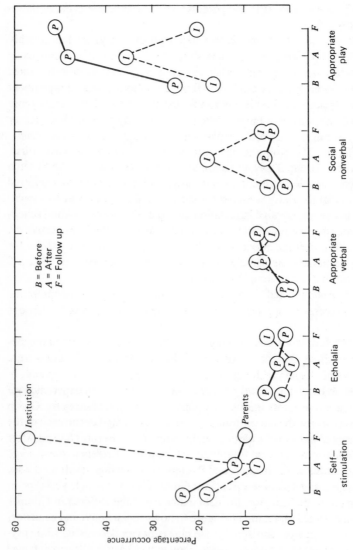

Figure 6. Percentage occurrence of multiple response measure behavioral categories for children whose parents were not trained in behavior modification (*I*) and for children whose parents were trained in behavior modification (*P*) before treatment (*B*), after treatment (*A*), and at follow-up (*F*). From O. I. Lovaas, R. Koegal, J. Q. Simmons, and J. Stevens-Long. Some generalization and followup measures on autistic children in behavior therapy, *Journal of Applied Behavior Analysis*, 1973, **6,** 131–166. Fig. 7. Copyright 1973 by the Society for the Experimental Analysis of Behavior, Inc.

(in Rick's case, 24 hours; for Pamela, three weeks). Multiple response recordings were obtained both before and after this intervention. The data show that even this short exposure to treatment was effective. All three appropriate behaviors increased, while self-stimulation decreased. The data suggest that the children had not forgotten what we had taught them, but their problem was essentially motivational.

More extensive presentation of the follow-up data may be found in Lovaas, *et al.* (1973). The findings consistently emphasize the point that, without therapeutically prescribed, functional reinforcement, children like these do not improve or retain whatever improvement they have made in treatment. The best way we know of to ensure a therapeutic post-treatment environment is to train parents in our procedures, and then to allow the parents to assume the role of primary therapist for their own child. We now consider it a mistake to hospitalize these children.

Finally, let us turn to the data on response generalization. Eighteen of the 20 children we have treated received Stanford-Binet Intelligence Scale tests before and after treatment; one child received the Merrill-Palmer. Fourteen of the 20 received the Vineland Social Maturity Scale. A summary of changes during treatment for intelligence test scores is presented in Figure 7. IQ scores are presented before *(B)* and *(A)* after treatment. Dotted lines indicate that the patient was untestable prior to treatment. Untestable means that the child could not respond appropriately to the examiner's attempts to test him. The children were often oblivious to the materials and requests presented to them. Most of the children, however, made substantial gains on the measures. Many who were untestable before our intervention were functioning at the mildly to moderately retarded level at termination of treatment. Some of the change in the untestable children reflects extinction of interfering behaviors; some reflects genuinely new acquisitions.

All of the 14 children for whom we have scores on the Vineland Social Maturity Scale showed large gains. The mean social quotient before treatment was 48 with a standard deviation of 20. The mean quotient after treatment was 71 with a standard deviation of 27. Again, much of this change was reflective of a reduction in bizarre behavior and the achievement of elementary social stimulus control. Again, there were no exceptions. All 14 of the children showed higher quotients after treatment than they had before treatment.

An extensive description of our attempts to provide data on reliability for the multiple response recordings may be found in Lovaas et al. (1973), where results are presented for two different methods of assessing reliability. Essentially, the data show a high degree of agreement between both experienced and naive Os, and the direction of change in treatment was the same whether recorded by a naive O or an experienced one. This is the case even when the pre- and post-treatment video-tape recordings of the measurement sessions are presented to a naive O in random order.

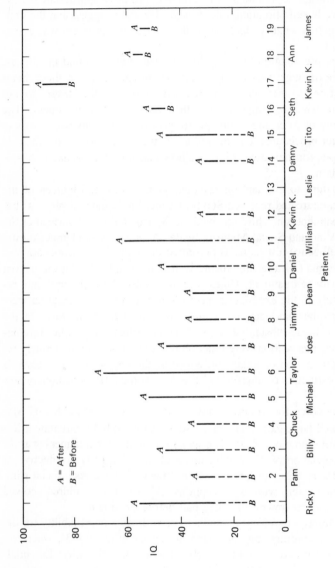

Figure 7. Intelligence quotients for 19 children. The names of the children appear on the abscissa and the IQ scores on the ordinate. Scores obtained before (*B*) and after (*A*) treatment are presented. Broken lines indicate that the child was considered untestable before treatment. From O. I. Lovaas, R. Koegal, J. Q. Simmons, and J. Stevens-Long, Some generalization and fol-lowup measures on autistic children in behavior therapy, *Journal of Applied Behavior Analysis*, 1973, **6**, 131–166, Fig. 9. Copyright 1973 by the Society for the Experimental Analysis of Behavior, Inc.

Probably one of the more pronounced features of our findings underscores casual observations that there is considerable heterogeneity in the degree of improvement shown by different children. Ricky might learn in one hour what Jose required one year to master. The major areas of improvement were not the same for each child. All of the parents reported gains in language and general attentiveness, but there was no systematic pattern with respect to the major areas of improvement reported.

The data from the measurement study, along with other observations presented in this review, have enabled us to draw some conclusions about our strengths and weaknesses as behavior modifiers. We appear to be particularly successful in suppressing self-destructive behavior. We have also been very good at rearranging behavior. For example, if a child was echolalic, then we could help him make large gains in language and intellectual behavior. Whatever gains the children made seemed to show at least some stimulus generalization. The behaviors the children acquired also indicate some response generalization, as the data on the IQ scores point out.

There were also some major disappointments. We failed to isolate a "pivotal" response; that is, we did not find one central behavior which, if altered, could effect profound "personality" changes. For example, we had once hoped that if the child learned his own name, awareness of "self," or some such development, would emerge. It did not. Perhaps behavior therapy is not the correct approach. But it is also possible that the problem is erroneously conceptualized. "Autism" may be a publicly and emotionally appealing term, but at this point it does not appear to indicate a common response to treatment. There may be no "pivotal" response.

It is also important to bear in mind that behavior therapy is a treatment based on research, rather than deduced from theory; therefore, it is constantly changing. Just a short time ago, many argued that children like those described here were unable to imitate and unable to form abstractions. Change does occur, but it seems to be of a gradual kind. We do not know all the functional relationships which might enable us to build a completely normal behavioral repertoire at this time, but we have taken a few steps and it is important to continue. To some extent, we are still trying to isolate the important issues. As we do isolate these issues, we can begin to define and test them. As an example of this process of definition and testing, let us turn to one of the most important current research problems being examined in our lab.

CURRENT RESEARCH

A number of questions continue to plague us in developing teaching programs for autistic children. Why do certain autistic children show much larger improvements than others? Why does a given autistic child show relatively large and rapid improvements in some areas and slow, minimal gains in other areas? Why do so few autistic children become normal?

Many researchers and clinicians have emphasized the extreme inconsistency with which autistic children respond to sensory input. This inconsistency and variability seemed to us to suggest deviant attentional behaviors; behaviors which might retard certain acquisitions. This line of reasoning led us to begin a series of studies designed to examine the possibility of attentional deviation more closely.

One of the earliest of these studies reports data for three groups of children, autistics, retardates, and normals (Lovaas, Kogel, Schreibman, & Rehm, 1971). All three groups were reinforced for responding when the experimenter *(E)* presented a complex stimulus involving auditory (five seconds of white noise), visual (a five-second red floodlight), and tactile (five seconds of pressure from a blood pressure cuff on *S*s calf) components. Once the child was reliably responding to the stimuli, 10 test sessions were arranged for each child to determine how he would respond to the stimuli if presented singly in random order.

The most general conclusion which can be drawn from the data collected in this study is that autistic children responded primarily to one stimulus component, retardates to two, and normals to all three. Subsequent training sessions showed that autistic children could learn to respond to the cues they did not respond to previously if the stimuli were presented for training individually. We argued on the basis of these results that autistic children do not show a "preference" for any one modality, or an impairment in any one modality. Instead, the children overselect modalities. To put it very simply, when they hear, they do not see, and when they see, they do not hear. Their behavior comes under the control of only a portion of the available stimuli.

These data suggested a number of ideas about learning in autistic children. A necessary condition for learning involves a contiguous, or nearly contiguous presentation of two stimuli. The development of appropriate affect, the acquisition of meaningful speech (at least as we have defined it), and the acquisition of secondary reinforcers, may all depend upon the child's learning about stimulus contiguity. When we attempt to teach the children appropriate behaviors like these, we usually proceed by adding extra cues (extra-stimulus prompts) to the training situation, or we pair two stimuli for the child (as in classical conditioning). This, of course, may be exactly what makes it so difficult for the autistic child to learn what we have set out to teach him. Thus the data on overselectivity have important implications for a training program such as ours. The work of Laura Schriebman (1973), described earlier in this review, expands upon the notion of stimulus overselectivity and begins to clarify how our training program might best be modified to allow for this attentional pattern.

SUMMARY

Over the period of the last 10 years, we have been able to demonstrate in a variety of ways that behavior modification is an effective procedure for changing the behavior of autistic children. This report summarizes these 10 years of data collection and therapy for 20 such children. The data for each child reflects measurable progress, although that progress was sometimes slow.

During these 10 years, much data was accumulated on a number of specific behaviors, and we learned more about some behaviors than others. We learned a great deal about self-destructive behavior. We were able to identify conditions which appear to control the behavior and to observe how changes in the consequences produced by self-destructive behavior result in changes in the frequency of the behavior. We did not learn as much about self-stimulation. The data show that the presence of self-stimulation makes it more difficult to teach a child and that self-stimulation appears to be maintained by reinforcers that compete with those that maintain other kinds of behavior. Beyond those limited observations, we know little about self-stimulation.

We have also established a fairly detailed set of procedures for teaching intellectual and social skills to autistic children and have presented a fair amount of data on the acquisition of a variety of skills including verbal imitation and labeling. Moreover, we have developed a system of measurement designed to assess more general changes in behavior during treatment. Findings from this more general assessment indicate that although every child gained something from the treatment program, we were of more help to some than to others. We were very good at rearranging behavior. For example, if the child exhibited verbal behavior before treatment, such as echolalic speech, we could help him develop meaningful language far more easily than we could establish verbal behavior in children who were mute.

The follow-up data presented here indicate that to maintain the gains made in treatment, the post-treatment environment must provide for therapeutically prescribed delivery of contingent, functional reinforcers. The best way we know of to ensure such a post-treatment environment is to train parents in the principles of behavior modification and allow them to assume primary responsibility for the child's treatment.

Over the years, it has become increasingly evident to us that these children exhibit important deviations in perceptual functioning. Currently, our research is directed at defining the parameters of the deficit and developing educational materials that will optimize learning given the problems these children show. The use of within-stimulus prompts is but one example of the ways in which our procedures may ultimately be revised by new research. Perhaps this is the most heartening aspect of the therapeutic framework we have adopted. Behavior modification not only allows for change in specific techniques and procedures, but it demands change. Where progress is slow or improvement limited, the underlying assumptions of the theory lead one to look for ways to improve treatment, to revise procedures, to change the environment. The theory is ultimately an extremely optimistic one. The assumption is always that behavior is modifiable, only our own ignorance prevents us from being of greater help.

REFERENCES

Allyon, T., & Azrin, N. H. The measurement and reinforcement of the behavior of psychotics. *Journal of the Experimental Analysis of Behavior.*, 1965, **8**, 357–383.

Baer, D. M., and Sherman, J. A. Reinforcement control of generalized imitation in young children. *Journal of Experimental Child Psychology*, 1964, **1**, 37–49.

Baer, D. M., Wolf, M. M., & Risley, T. R. Some current dimensions of applied behavior analysis. *Journal of Applied Behavior Analysis*, 1968, **1**, 91–97.

Brackbill, Y., Adams, G., Crowell, D. H., & Gray, M. L. Arousal level in neonates and preschool children under continuous auditory stimulation. *Journal of Experimental Child Psychology*, 1966, **4**, 178–188.

Ferster, C. B. Positive reinforcement and behavioral deficits of autistic children. *Child Development*, 1961, **32**, 437–456.

Hayes, C. *The ape in our house.* New York: Harper, 1951.

Hermelin, B. Recent psychological research. In J. K. Wing (Ed.), *Early childhood autism.* London: Pergamon Press, 1966.

Isaacs, W., Thomas, J., & Goldiamond, I. Application of operant conditioning to reinstate verbal behavior in psychotics. *Journal of Speech and Hearing Disorders*, 1960, **25**, 8–15.

Kanner, L., & Eisenberg, L. Early infantile autism. *Psychiatric Research Report*, 1957, **1**, 55–65.

Koegel, R. Selective attention to prompt stimuli by autistic and normal children. Unpublished doctoral dissertation, University of California, Los Angeles, 1971.

Koegel, R., & Wilhelm, H. Selective responding to multiple visual cues by autistic children. *Journal of Experimental Child Psychology*, in press.

Lovaas, O. I. Behavior therapy approach to the treatment of childhood schizophrenia. In J. Hill (Ed.), *Minnesota symposium on child development.* Minneapolis; University of Minnesota Press, 1967.

Lovaas, O. I. Teaching language to non-linguistic children. Unpublished manuscript, 1973.

Lovaas, O. I., Berberich, J. P., Perloff, B. F., & Schaeffer, B. Acquisition of imitative speech by schizophrenic children. *Science*, 1966, **151**, 705–707.

Lovaas, O. I., Freitag, G., Gold, V. J., & Kassorla, I. C. Experimental studies in childhood schizophrenia: Analysis of self-destructive behavior. *Journal of Experimental Child Psychology*, 1965, **2**, 67–84.

Lovaas, O. I., Freitag, G., Kinder, M. I., Rubenstein, B. D., Schaeffer, B., & Simmons, J. Q. Establishment of social reinforcers in schizophrenic children using food. *Journal of Experimental Child Psychology*, 1966, **4**, 109–125.

Lovaas, O. I., Koegel, R., Simmons, J. Q., & Stevens-Long, J. Some generalization and follow-up measures on autistic children in behavior therapy. *Journal of Applied Behavior Analysis*, 1973, **6**, 131–166.

Lovaas, O. I., Litronik, A., & Mann, R. Response latencies to auditory stimuli in autistic children engaged in self-stimulatory behavior. *Behavior Research and Therapy*, 1971, **9**, 39–50.

Lovaas, O. I., & Schreibman, L. Stimulus overselectivity of autistic children in a two stimulus situation. *Behavior Research and Therapy*, 1971, **2**, 305–310.

Lovaas, O. I., Schreibman, L., Koegel, R., & Rehm, R. Selective responding by autistic children to multiple sensory input. *Journal of Abnormal Psychology*, 1971, **77**, 211–222.

Lovaas, O. I., & Simmons, J. Q. Manipulation of self destruction in three retarded children. *Journal of Applied Behavior Analysis*, 1969, **2**, 143–157.

O'Leary, R. D., & Drabman, R. Token economy programs in the classroom: A Review. *Psychological Bulletin*, 1971, **75**, 379–398.

Rimland, B. *Infantile autism*. New York: Appleton-Century-Crofts, 1964.

Risley, T. R. The establishment of verbal behavior in deviant children. Unpublished doctoral dissertation, University of Washington, Seattle, 1966.

Risley, T. R. The effects and side effects of punishing the autistic behaviors of a deviant child. *Journal of Applied Behavior Analysis*, 1968, **1**, 21–34.

Schreibman, L. Within-stimulus versus extra-stimulus prompting procedures in discriminations with autistic children. Unpublished doctoral dissertation, University of California, Los Angeles, 1972.

Sherman, J. A. Use of reinforcement and imitation to reinstate verbal behavior in mute psychotics. *Journal of Abnormal Psychology*, 1965, **70**, 155–164.

Skinner, B. F. *Verbal behavior*. New York: Appleton-Century-Crofts, 1957.

Stone, A. A. Consciousness: Altered levels in blind retarded children. *Psychosomatic Medicine*, 1964, **26**, 14–19.

Thompson, T., & Grabowski, J. (Eds.). *Behavior modification of the mentally retarded*. New York: Oxford University Press, 1972.

Thorp, R. G., & Wetzel, R. J. *Behavior modification in the natural environment*. New York: Academic Press, 1969.

Wasserman, L. M. Discrimination learning in autistic children. Unpublished doctoral dissertation, University of California, Los Angeles, 1968.

Wolf, M., Risley, T. R., & Mees, H. Application of operant conditioning procedures to the behavior problems of an autistic child. *Behavior Research and Therapy*, 1964, **1**, 305–312.

Wolpe, J. *Psychotherapy by reciprocal inhibition*. Stanford, California: University of Stanford Press, 1958.

Wolpe, J. *The practice of behavior therapy*. Elmsford, N. Y.: Pergamon Press, 1969.

CHAPTER 6

Changes of Direction with Psychotic Children

ERIC SCHOPLER

The most puzzling of childhood disorders to have appeared in psychiatric clinics has been childhood psychosis or autism. Clinicians have used other names for these children, but the proliferation of diagnostic terms has done little to diminish anyone's puzzlement. On the contrary, it is fair to say that low diagnostic consensus among clinicians correlates significantly with low scientific knowledge available to date. The combination of unsubstantiated beliefs and the pressure to answer clinical questions have resulted in substantial confusion, especially in parents and others charged with the decisions of dealing with these youngsters.

Since the formal introduction of autism in the psychiatric literature only three decades ago (Kanner, 1943), there has been a noticeable shift from the global generalizations of psychoanalytic thinking to more specific information from current research. This chapter traces some of the sources of past confusion, including the shift from theoretical beliefs to more empirically based information. This shift is traced through *(a)* classification, *(b)* theories of causation, *(c)* role of parents, *(d)* treatment interventions, and *(e)* social and ecological considerations. In each of these areas the writer attempts to summarize the current state of affairs and to hazard a projection of future trends based on his own research and clinical experience.

HISTORICAL BACKGROUND

Children similar to those who might today be called psychotic or autistic have been reported far back in human history. These children, and even the term au-

Both research and treatment approaches discussed in this chapter were formulated in collaboration with Robert J. Reichler. The scope of his contribution to both over the past seven years cannot be detailed, but is gratefully acknowledged.

tism, have been shrouded by myth and mystique. Reports of wild, feral children, reared by wolves and other animals, trace back to early Roman history. It is of some interest that the most recent published report of children raised by wolves, and the first mention of autistic children, should fall within three years of each other. No less eminent a physician than Arnold Gesell (1941) accepted the credibility of wolves rearing human children. More recently Bettelheim (1959) published a refutation of the existence of feral children. Instead he submitted clinical evidence suggesting to him that feral children were actually autistic. While he rejected the existence of feral children, he substituted the existence of feral mothers as the primary sources of autistic development.

From this intersection between autistic and feral children, we attempt to obtain some insight into the primitive confusion and suspension of rationality which still characterizes some approaches to severely disturbed children even today. For the purpose of this review some parallel lapses of rationality in both Gesell and Bettelheim are reviewed.

In "Wolf Child and Human Child," Gesell reviews the diary kept by Reverend Singh of his observations and experiences in rearing two feral children from October 8, 1920, to November 14, 1929, at which time the second of the two feral children died at age 17. The Rev. Singh presumably reclaimed both of these children from a wolf's den, one of the children then being eight years old. Dr. Gesell's fascination with the Singh diary is readily understood. Here was an extreme example of the nature-nurture problem he had been concerned with throughout his professional career. He had achieved great distinction for his painstaking observations and recordings of developmental sequences characterizing the age levels of normal children. In Singh's diary Gesell found evidence that these feral, Indian children raised by wolves, went through some of the same developmental sequences that he had discovered in the largest sample of his researches, that is, the middle class population of New Haven. On the face of it, this finding may not be too surprising. However, his unquestioning acceptance of their presumed foster care by wolves and his interpretation of the children's deviant behavior as normal are nothing less than amazing.

Any scientific or rational reflection on the effects of wolf foster parents on human children might begin with the credibility for the existence of their interaction. Could and would wolves raise human children rather than eat them? What was the evidence for the belief that wolves would rear children over extended periods, and who reported the evidence? Gesell asked none of these questions. The accounts of this phenomenon came to him twice removed—first reported by Rev. Singh in India and second translated by Dr. Zingg in Denver. Gesell did not acknowledge that the translation may have taken a toll in the accuracy of the original. Moreover, he passed without question any possible bias and distortions in Singh's story. By his own report, the Rev. Singh was a missionary with a zeal for seeking out primitive tribes for conversion. In one village the natives had been terrified by wild, ghost children. Singh dispelled these ghosts by discovering that they were actually children raised by wolves. Instead of at least examining the spiritual or miraculous context of the children's discovery, Gesell blithely reconstructed what their life was like in the wolf den and how the wolf culture affected their development.

Even more astonishing than Gesell's unscientific acceptance of hearsay with superimposed fiction is his treatment of claims that these feral children were "normal." Gesell stated (1941, p. 72) that when Kamalar was 17 years old her language and social behavior was that of a three-year-old child. Nevertheless, ". . . the available evidence strongly denotes that Kamula was born a normal infant . . ." and that she suffered no disease or injury that would destroy the normal potentialities of her brain. In fact Gesell noted that (1941, p. 73), "There are significant clinical indications of her essential normality." The indications cited by Gesell include Kamula's successful adjustment to the wolf den, an adjustment which had in fact been reconstructed purely from Gesell's imagination (1941, pp. 9–13).

In the paragraphs above I have tried to show how a contemporary myth was created. A child clearly described as functioning on a mentally deficient level can be considered normal because she was raised by wolves. A second myth, more directly related to the treatment of autistic children, was propagated by Bettelheim (1959). He also disbelieved that the children raised by Singh were reared by wolves. He referred to Ogburn's successful proof that there was no sound evidence of animal foster parents (without reference). He believed that these wild children could not have survived wilderness conditions very long by themselves, even allowing for the clemency of Indian weather. Instead, he presented convincing examples that feral children behaved very much like autistic children at his school. He argued that the so-called feral children were actually autistic children who had been neglected and emotionally deprived by their mothers. Bettelheim claimed that by correcting this widely held error on the origins of feral children, he may have contributed more to social science than with the discovery of any new theory. He concluded that he had succeeded in demonstrating that there are no feral children, but perhaps only feral mothers. With this conclusion he promoted a most pervasive and harmful myth regarding the causes of autism.

Two of the myths propogated by Bettelheim and Gesell in explanation of legendary feral children have been detrimental to the understanding of autistic or psychotic children. These include Gesell's caricature definition of "normal" as human behavior that may be acceptable in a wolf's den, and Bettelheim's revelation that there were no feral children. Instead they were autistic children with feral mothers. Both myths emerged from an era when nature versus nurture was simplistically dichotemized. Human biology was regarded as primarily fixed and developmental deviations were mainly considered as reactions to extremes in the external environment.

More current explanations of the feral child phenomenon would stress that some appeared to have at least normal functions. Romulus and Remus were apparently able to found Rome after being set adrift on the Tiber. Kasper Hauser was able to make us his educational deficits after 17 years in a solitary dungeon. However, most others, like Dina Sanicher, the wolf child of Sikandra, Victor, the Wild Boy of Averyon, and Rev. Singh's Kamula all had unknown periods of abandonment and also suffered varying degrees of retardation.

We now recognize that a poor human environment with deficiencies in diet and basic care can also predispose to genetic and biological maldevelopment. We have become increasingly interested in clarifying more specific effects of biological, psychological, and environmental interactions on a child's development, for example, the interaction between neonatal nutrition, biological structures, and intelligence. There is now also greater awareness that these interaction patterns vary with the child's level of development. For example, the biological structures involving bowel control have a greater effect on the child's interaction with his mother during early childhood than they will at older age levels. Likewise, an autistic child's biological impairment makes his child–parent interactions less reciprocal than would normal biological functions. The interaction is determined from the needs created by the impairment rather than only by normal needs.

It would appear that some social science conceptions are readily extrapolated into developmental mythology. Enemies of normal development may be identified as wolves, as feral mothers, or as deficient biological structures in the child. We should not, however, be too concerned over the links between science and myth. The intellectual absurdities and social harm stem far less from sound myths than from the human tendency to persist with theoretical positions and conclusions at the cost of ignoring new data. This is a similar tendency to making unlimited generalizations from limited data or experience. In this chapter, an attempt is made to identify historical excesses of belief and theories, some of which still persist; to select research and clinical data which are consistent with new directions of understanding and treatment of autistic children; and to mark guidelines for avoiding the excesses obvious in the past and so elusive in the present efforts to affect the future.

CLASSIFICATION

Perhaps the most clearly defined of the terms representing severely disturbed children has been infantile autism. It was formulated in 1943 when Kanner reported on a series of children he had examined at Johns Hopkins. His definition was translatably succinct and soon children with similar symptoms were described in the psychiatric literature of other clinics and countries. During this period numerous other diagnostic terms referring to severely disturbed children appeared. Some of these terms were characterized by a prominent clinician's name and his distinct theoretical position. Childhood schizophrenia was the term used by Bender (1953). She believed these children suffered from impairments in various biological functions to which the child responded with schizophrenic anxiety. Mahler (1952) introduced symbiotic psychosis with the key explanation referring to the mother's anxiety preventing her young child from separating and individuating himself. Other diagnostic terms might best be characterized by the geographic area from which the investigator reported. Rank (1950) introduced the atypical child in the Boston area, while Ekstein (1954) at Menninger's formulated borderline psychosis. Yet other labels such as primary disorders of childhood and minimal brain damage helped cloud the clinical arena. No consensus has developed among clinicians as to how these diagnostic labels differentiate children from each other. This confusion of terminology has hampered the treatment of psychotic or autistic children and limited the applicability of research findings from one clinic to another. The basis of the confusion may be found in the limits of actual knowledge about psychosis and in problems inherent in the classification process.

There are numerous valid criteria for identifying classification categories. For example, a group of objects can be subdivided by color, by shape, by function, by smell, and so on. The particular criteria used depend on the purposes for classifying the objects in the first place. In the case of psychiatric disorders there are three major bases for diagnostic classification: (1) One or more specific cause(s) are known for the disorder, as for example with phenylketonuria. In the case of autism or psychosis, no such specific causes are known. (2) A specific treatment exists, applicable to one group of children, but not others. For autism or childhood psychosis some success has been reported for many different treatments; therefore, this second basis does not apply either. (3) Certain behaviors and observable characteristics can be identified and described. Current efforts with diagnostic classification are mainly at this third level. Some behaviorists have concluded from this state of affairs that there is no use to any classification except behavior. They would argue, for example, that a normal child isolated in an empty room will show self-stimulating behavior much like an autistic child in a back ward. Yet the two children in this example will obviously appear different. Such diagnostic nihilism ignores the little knowledge that is available and also precludes the development of more meaningful classification based on increased knowledge.

Description of Childhood Psychosis

An important step out of this labeling morass was taken by Creak (1964) and the working party of clinicians that she directed. They set themselves the task of identifying common characteristics of children with the different diagnostic labels mentioned above. From these discussions emerged nine criteria. These nine points were behaviorally oriented and mostly quite specific.

These points included the following:

1. Gross and sustained impairment of emotional relationships with people. This indicated aloofness, excessive clinging, and other outstanding and lasting relationship difficulties.

2. Unawareness of his own personal identity. This could be seen in peculiar posturing, and self-directed aggression.

3. Pathological preoccupation with certain objects without regard to their accepted functions.

4. Sustained resistance to change in the environment and striving to maintain sameness.

5. Abnormal perceptual experience, as the diminished, excessive, or unpredictable response to sensory stimuli—for example, visual or auditory avoidance, and insensitivity to pain and temperatures.

6. Frequent, acute, and excessive anxiety that seemed illogical to the observer.

7. Speech may have been lost or never acquired, or may have failed to develop beyond a level appropriate to an earlier age. There may be confusion of personal pronouns, echolalia, and other mannerisms of speech and diction. Words and phrases may be used, but without appropriate meaning.

8. Distortion in motility patterns such as hyperactivity or hypoactivity, ritualistic mannerisms, rocking and spinning.

9. A background of serious retardation in which islets of near normal or exceptional intellectual function or skill may appear.

These nine points still presented some problems for reliability of ratings. However, they also offered increased clarity and agreement for comparing children from one place to another. Although the Creak criteria included most of the behaviors described by Kanner for infantile autism, they also included a wider spectrum of behavior, thus broadening the Kanner definition. Accordingly, the terms autism and childhood psychosis are used interchangeably in this discussion.

A second recent step in improving current methods of classifications was suggested by the World Health Organization. The methodological contribution from this group (Rutter, 1972) came from their recognition that certain dimensions in the child's condition required separate assessment. In this multiaxial classification system, four axes were suggested.

The first specified the clinical psychiatric syndrome; the second, the intellectual level; the third, any associated or etiological biological factors; and the fourth, any associated or etiological psychosocial factors.

According to Rutter, this system had the advantages of avoiding the most common disagreement among clinicians—causational emphasis of the diagnosis. For example, if a psychotic child with mild retardation has epileptic fits, each of these three axes can be evaluated separately, without needing to decide whether the epilepsy caused the psychosis, was a secondary contributory factor, or the other way around. After all, Rutter concluded, meaningful communication between clinicians of different theoretical persuasions is what classification is all about.

Future Trends in Classification

Using a multiaxial classification method, it is possible that a more scientific and practical application can be developed than the one suggested by Rutter. Possibly to allow communication between clinicians who have convictions about primary causes based on their varying theoretical persuasions may not be the most scientific purpose. It may make for more harmonious psychiatric and clinical conferences, even on an international scale, but this is not necessarily the same as improving the treatment and understanding of severely disturbed children. On the contrary, neither classification of a child nor communications about his behavior disorders can be any better than what is actually known about his disorder. At this time, for almost any individual psychotic child, we do not know the specific causes of his disorder with adequate certainty. The substitution of theoretical persuasions for this uncertainty is often counterproductive clinically and it is certainly not scientific.

Perhaps the main guiding purpose of future classification will shift from communication among professionals to making possible the most appropriate decision regarding each severely disturbed child. In the absence of adequate knowledge, multiple axes may still be needed. But rather than considering each category as discrete or absolute, an interaction system could be developed. Under the World Health Organization system the first axis specified the clinical psychiatric syndrome. This could be elaborated to include not only the direction of a behavioral symptom but also the circumstances. For example, an autistic youngster may be reported as showing self-destructive head-banging while left on his own in a custodial day care program, but he does not show this behavior during a structured teaching period at home. On the second axis, instead of citing a child's IQ or intellectual level, a learning profile could be substituted. This would include a breakdown of his various mental functions and the developmental levels achieved in each area. Thus a child may show a verbal level of three years, a gross motor level of six years, and self-help skills at a four-year level, and so on. The third axis of biological factors could include not only the evidence for the kind and scope of biological impairment, but also the biochemical interventions which are likely or have been tried, and the effects of the trials. The fourth axis of etiological psychosocial factors may be replaced by an environmental evaluation profile. For the child's family this would include their resources, financially, emotionally, and intellectually for coping with the child's special problems. For their community, it would include the relevant resources of special education, day care, medical supervision, speech and hearing assessment, and so on. This system would be somewhat more elaborate and cumbersome than the diagnostic systems proposed by various medical groups. However, this would be a small price to pay for the usual and often cruel gap between diagnosis and what to do about it.

FACTORS OF CAUSATION

In the previous section I tried to trace the past chaos and confusion of diagnostic labeling to some of the more rational efforts of the last decade. This diagnostic confusion seems best explained by the absence of scientific knowledge of specific causes. Historically, coping with the unknown frequently fell into the province of theology. During the past century this struggle was increasingly carried on in the medical domain. This resulted in some scientific gains but also in the substitution of misleading theories for admission of the unknown. One of the most pervasive and best known of the psychiatric theories is the psychoanalytically derived notion that parental attitudes, emotions, and psychopathologies are the main cause for autistic or psychotic development in their child.

When Kanner (1943) first wrote on infantile autism, he referred to the constitutional predisposition to autistic development in the child. However, he also described the parents of these children as uniquely obsessive, intellectual, uncreative, and emotionally cold (Kanner, 1949). It is to Kanner's lasting credit that in the absence of research findings he recognized the interaction between biological factors in the child and his environment. However, the main emphasis in clinical practice remained clearly on the effects of parental attitudes and personality characteristics. There was an overwhelming tendency to regard parental emotional responses as the main cause for the child's autistic, social, and emotional withdrawal from a hostile world.

Changes in the current views of the underlying factors in autism are traced for three of the major symptoms of impairment. These include the disturbance in human relatedness, the uneven and retarded intellectual functions, and the inability to use appropriate language.

Disturbance of Human Relatedness

Although there has been little agreement among clinicians about the meaning of various diagnostic terms introduced during the past three decades, there was some noticeable consensus on one point. Whether a child was tagged psychotic, schizophrenic, atypical, or autistic, it was usually agreed that he also suffered from disturbed human relationships. This symptom, like some of the others, was explained in terms of the inadequacies discovered by clinicians in the dynamics of family relationships.

In the current perspective, inadequacies in the child's social interaction are still recognized. However, research efforts have made it possible to move from the global to the more discrete. It has become increasingly evident that human relatedness is based on a degree of intact perceptual, language, and intellectual functions, missing with varying degress in psychotic children. Their perceptual peculiarities had been observed in the past (Goldfarb, 1956; Schopler, 1965). A series of studies by Ornitz (1968) demonstrated that the inability to maintain constancies of perception was an underlying difficulty for psychotic children. In a similar vein, Reichler and Schopler (1971) conducted a factor analytic study of children seen in the Child Research Project, a program for psychotic children and their parents. In this study, 64 children were rated on 14 diagnostic scales based on the Creak (1964) criteria. Factor 1 identified by the analysis referred to human relations. A multiple regression analysis was made of variables significant at the earlier levels of development. We found that perceptual variables such as near receptor, auditory, and visual responsiveness all were highly predictive of the human relatedness factor. Even a cautious interpretation of these findings would suggest that it is less parsimonious to regard impairments in human relatedness as a primary causal effect of other perceptual functions. Instead it would appear that the impairments in a child's perceptual systems would be bound to make for impairment in his human relationships.

These research findings were also consistent with frequently reported clinical observations. That is, as the underlying incongruities of perception, language, and intellectual function are either remedied or accepted, psychotic children tended to become less aloof and more affectionate (Wing, 1972).

Uneven and Retarded Intellectual Functions

As has already been noted under the early global explanation, the autistic child's primary defect in relatedness was considered a disturbance in affective contact (Kanner, 1943). The child appeared mentally retarded because of his social withdrawal. These children were widely believed to have normal intellectual potential. If the youngster happened to have some isolated skills, such as musical memory or memory for dates, coupled with an inability to take care of himself, then such peak skills were regarded as evidence of his normal intellectual potential. When no support for this view could be found from psychological testing, the negative result was explained away as the "untestability" of these children. Poor motivation, interpersonal avoidance, and lack of cooperation were the most common explanations for the child's "untestability."

More systematic research efforts have suggested a different line of reasoning (Alpern, 1967; Gittelman & Birch, 1967). An autistic child may be untestable because the wrong tests are used. Projective tests are usually not helpful. They require language skills and conceptual thinking, often unavailable to psychotic children. They also try to answer psychoanalytic questions, which are usually inappropriate to psychotic children. Other tests, like the Binet, rely almost completely on understanding spoken language, and thus heighten the barrier to mental assessment. But even when more appropriate tests are used, like the Leiter International, the Merrill-Palmer, the Bayley, tests that do not rely mainly on language skills, the child may still appear "untestable" and unresponsive. Alpern has shown that autistic children who were uncooperative at one developmental test level of a test did respond to easier or earlier developmental test items. If the child completes an easier test item, he cannot be considered simply uncooperative or withdrawn. If he were, he would not answer the easier items either. According to the withdrawal view, the autistic child would function normally if his affective negativism could be neutralized, or if some past environmental trauma could be relived. In other words, the dynamics of his emotional withdrawal are regarded as the main reason for his lack of response to the test items. Current evidence suggests that psychotic children are most negative in those areas in which they have the most impairment. They usually have more difficulty with using and understanding language than they do with motor skills. Likewise, they show more avoidance and negativism with language than motor activities.

As the concept of untestability has faded in current programs for psychotic children, variability in the psychotic child's response to psychological testing has become more apparent. The recently discovered testability of these children has shown that their IQ scores are often at a lower level than the social withdrawal beliefs allowed us to recognize. This new knowledge should not surprise anyone. IQ scores do tend to correlate with the verbal skills needed for adequate social adaptation, and this is a recognized central handicap in childhood psychosis.

The currently more successful testing procedures with these children show clearer retardation and impairment through what was previously considered the veil of autism or "untestability." Could this clearer awareness go against the best interest of the children? Their parents may become discouraged and give up on trying to help them. Many well-meaning clinicians have expressed this concern. Our experience has been in the opposite direction. Parents are spared the stress of false hopes for clearing away autism as an emotional problem. The children are spared the stress that comes from denying the needed acceptance of their intellectual impairment.

Language Function

The language impairment of autistic children takes on various forms. These range from absence of speech to speech delay, nonsense sentences, playing with words and phrases without meaning, echolalia or repetition of the last word heard, and pronoun reversal. The language problem of such children does not include, to any significant extent, withholding of language. They do not show a deliberate avoidance of intact speech, sometimes referred to as elective mutism. They do not usually express higher language skills away from their parents as might be expected if they were withdrawing from rejecting and emotionally cold social interaction.

According to the global withdrawal explanation, Bettelheim (1967) asserted that the child's lack of normal speech was in reaction to unresponsive parents who induced the kind of extreme hopelessness and negativism found in inmates of concentration camps. In addition to creating this metaphor of motivational extreme, Bettelheim argued that speech peculiarities such as pronoun reversal were caused by the child's lack of personal identity. Lack of supporting evidence has made this kind of psychological explanation virtually obsolete. There are children who have suffered extreme deprivation, of having their parents beat and break their bodies, as in the battered baby syndrome. Such children have not been reported as autistic. Moreover, autistic children usually have normal siblings by the same parents.

The idea that pronoun reversal represented lack of identity has also been superseded. This speech peculiarity is often the same as echolalia. That is, the child repeats the last words heard including pronouns. The learning of pronouns also requires more complex mental activity than is often recognized. For example, in teaching correct pronoun usage by saying, "Show me that *your* eyes are reading these words," if you point at *your* eyes, in fact you could be demonstrating *my* eyes. You could then point to *my* eyes, but you could also be demonstrating *your* eyes. Obviously correct use depends on from whose point of view the pronoun is articulated. With one autistic child we were able to demonstrate (Schopler & Reichler, 1969) that correct pronoun usage could be taught more rapidly if the pronoun property of reversability was removed from the teaching situation. This was done by practicing pronoun usage with the child in a circle including the teacher, a male doll, a female doll, and the child. The use of these figures helped to stabilize pronouns, and the autistic youngster replaced pronoun reversal with correct usage within a two-week period.

Generally speaking, autistic children who reverse pronouns often also have difficulty with other equally complex concepts. The difficulty of understanding is basic to autism (Wing, 1972). It has been demonstrated as an impairment in integrating sensory information (Ornitz, 1968; Schopler, 1966) as well as understanding language (Rutter, 1968).

In summary, on the basis of the most current reviews (Rutter, 1968; Ornitz, 1973) certain statements may be proposed regarding the causes of autism: (1) the causes are multiply determined; (2) in individual cases the specific causes are usually unknown; and (3) most likely the primary causes involve some form of brain abnormality, including impairment of age appropriate perception and understanding. The resulting variability in behavioral symptoms depends in large part on the child's age, the time of onset, and the severity of the impairment.

Future Trends

With continued research, especially in genetics, biochemistry, and neurobiology, the prospects are good for identifying clearer relationships between impairment of biological structures and behavioral abnormalities.

That is not to say that there is any realistic hope of clearing up autism or childhood psychosis by discovering a genetic, metabolic, or biochemical cause. However, from the relatively large and undifferentiated groups of psychotic children, it is possible to identify subclusters of children who share specific causal mechanisms for their psychotic behavior. As such subgroups are identified, they will also add to the small core of meaningful diagnostic terms.

PARENTS OF AUTISTIC CHILDREN

One of the most far-reaching errors in the relatively short time autism has been in the psychiatric literature has been the part ascribed to parents by mental health professionals for the development of the autistic child's disabilities. Parents have been regarded as the primary causative agents for their child's "psychotic," "autistic," "schizophrenic," or "symbiotic" development. In spite of the central role assigned to parents, they were not given the same clinical and diagnostic care lavished on their children. Instead they were characterized by homey epithets such as "emotionally cold," "rejecting," "refrigerator mothers," "smothering mothers"; and by pseudoscientific jargon like "schizophrenic," "overintellectual," "obsessive compulsive," and "feral mothers." With the exception of coining creative labels, those committed to the psychogenic theory, placing the etiologic emphasis on parental thought and feeling, have generated virtually no substantiating research nor empirical data to help explain the specific processes involved in autism (Rutter, 1968). Instead they have contributed to clinical practices and attitudes bearing striking similarities to the mechanisms of scapegoating (Allport, 1966; Schopler, 1971).

All three degrees of scapegoating identified by Allport can be found in the professionals occupying the field of mental health. The mildest degree may be a simple preference—for children versus parents, for the neurotically normal rather than the severely disturbed child. The second degree involving stereotyped, hard to change prejudices, is equally common. Manifestations include clinical evaluations in which children's pathology is consistently interpreted as a function of parental personality and character. Any ambiguous clinical evidence is interpreted with the perception that parental pathology was the primary agent in the child's adjustment problem. The third stage refers to overt acts of scapegoating. These are not based on an individual's intrinsic qualities, but on a "label" branding the individual with undesirable characteristics or as belonging to a discredited group. Even when parents have not regarded themselves as "patients," they have been asked to submit themselves to "intensive psychotherapy" if their child is to be seen; or they have been told that the only hope for their child is a complete and permanent separation from them (Bettelheim, 1967).

Various motivations for scapegoating parents are built into the professional structure of mental health clinicians. These include the following.

1. *Frustration*   The diagnostic confusion and lack of specific knowledge of causes and remedies place a frustrating burden on the clinician whose specialized training and expert role makes ignorance in his field frustrating to deal with.

2. *Guilt evasion*   Since the clinician's role includes turning knowledge into practice, the absence of adequate information may be experienced as guilt. The resulting anger is less readily discharged against autistic children than against their parents.

3. *Self-enhancement*   Since the autistic child is often unrelated, unresponsive, and slow to learn, the clinician is threatened with a sense of inferiority and failure. When his expert role is threatened and he is working within a system that requires him to charge a high fee for his time, he is under pressure to rationalize his role. The already existing traces of guilt, insecurity, and desperation in the parents form a convenient handle for trying to explain and rectify the plight of both child and clinician. The parents' perplexity is readily interpreted as a primary cause for the psychosis.

4. *Conformity*   When the predominant orientation of the clinic is the psychogenic view, then the emphasis on parental pathology for explaining children's difficulties is a shared belief among the staff. The senior staff's working assumptions are reinforced by a wide array of social sanctions.

5. *Tabloid thinking* (or the need for simplification).   In a case of childhood psychosis, the clinician is often confronted with a staggering array of potentially significant factors. These can include organic problems with hard and soft signs; unusual sensory and perceptual processes in the child; possible effects of potentially traumatic experiences; genetic taint; dietary and glandular deficits; irregular intellectual functions; guilty, perplexed, and exhausted parents—to name some of the more prominent factors for consideration. Their appropriate evaluation is usually difficult, time consuming, and incomplete. Critical thought is

more easily replaced by simplifications and tabloid thinking, or by cliches and labels.

These motivational explanations are plausible, but they are not as well established as the scapegoating-of-parents phenomenon itself. Parental and scientific indignation against these biases has been published with increased frequency in recent years (Rimland, 1964; Eberhardy, 1967; Kysar, 1968; Park, 1967; Schopler, 1971; Pitfield & Oppenheim, 1964). Some of these include parents' personal accounts of distressing treatment by various professionals they encountered while searching for help with their child. These experiences are both convincing and disturbing. Here are parents whose families are under special stress for trying to cope with their psychotic child and his special handicaps. Rather than finding either social supports or some sympathetic enlightenment, these families had both their guilt and confusion increased. It may be argued that these were individual cases whose experiences may have been unique or even distorted. However, certain studies of parents with psychotic children highlight problems they had in common as a group.

Two studies from our Center were selected which involved parents directly in a controlled experiment to allow for relatively more objectivity than is possible with individual case studies. In the two issues selected we examined the widely held belief (1) that parents of psychotic children suffer from thought disorders themselves, and (2) that parents of psychotic children misperceive their own child.

Do Parents Suffer from Thought Disorders?

This question has been examined with the use of the Goldstein-Scherer Object Sorting Test (OST) on several occasions during recent years. During this period, clinical investigators described the emotional expressions, ideas, and personalities of parents in intriguing parallels to their psychotic offspring. Parents' aberrant thinking was linked to the thought structures found in their schizophrenic offsprings (Wild, 1965; Lidz, 1958; Singer & Wynne, 1965) and a causal relationship was inferred. The studies using the OST were done with parents of adult schizophrenics and no distinction was made by age of onset, a distinction which has more recently been accepted as differentiating psychotic children from schizophrenic adults (Rutter, 1972).

The measure of disordered thinking in these parents was their response to the Object Sorting Test (OST). This test is simply a miscellaneous assortment of objects, both real (a bicycle bell) and play (toy screwdriver), including different shapes, colors, and functions. The task is to put together those objects which go together and to explain why they do. These explanations are then scored and rated according to a reasonably reliable and useable method developed by Lovibond (1954).

We (Schopler & Loftin, 1969) anticipated that parents of psychotic children would show less impaired thinking in their responses than did the parents of adult schizophrenics reported in other studies. This was not, however, what we found. A x^2 analysis showed that there were no significant differences in the impairment scores reported in the four studies we compared.

This negative finding was more surprising and perhaps even more interesting than if our expected hypothesis had been upheld. We were now forced to reconsider the study and to find whether the unexpected finding could be explained in terms of research design, data collection, or sample. All 34 parents in our study had been located at a traditional, psychoanalytically oriented clinic where they had been bringing their psychotic children for psychotherapy. The parents were required to be seen for psychotherapy themselves as well as were their children.

It occurred to us that any testing of parents done in the context of a psychogenic treatment program could be quite threatening and anxiety-producing for them. They already sensed that the clinical staff was disposed to attributing peculiarities in the child to parental personality characteristics. Parents may have been concerned that their OST would confirm and formalize their guilt. While the other studies using the OST did not specify the context of their testing, perhaps a similar "experimentally induced" test anxiety was also evoked in those parents.

To check this question, we located a second sample of parents. This group was not to be involved in any conjoint therapy with their children at the time of testing. In addition, as in the previous sample, the children were to have a psychiatric diagnosis of childhood psychosis or autism and to show at least four out of the nine signs for psychosis formulated by Creak. We already knew that the large majority of psychotic or autistic children had normal siblings. This meant that the majority of parents also had experienced normal parent–child interactions. We could now devise a testing context in which parents were interviewed about their successful child rearing experiences, instead of worrying them with their feelings of failure about their psychotic youngsters.

A standard interview was devised for questioning parents along the theme: How did you manage to succeed in raising a normal child with the presence of a problem child in the family? Parents were then asked to relate their success in disciplining and rewarding, encouraging school work, friendships, and family cooperation in their normal children. Needless to say, they all became involved in this interview, enjoyed supplying the information, and felt good about their parent role. They were given the OST after these interviews were completed. The resulting scores were compared with the scores from two sets of control parents, those with normal children and those with retarded children.

As anticipated, we found that parents tested in the context of psychogenically oriented therapy for their psychotic child obtained higher thought impairment scores than did parents of retarded and of normal children. Parents who were tested in the context of their successful child-rearing experiences did not differ significantly from the control parents of normal and retarded children. These findings clearly suggested that there was no evidence for a formal thought disorder in parents of psychotic children. Instead, their test scores appeared to be responsive to the presence or absence of situation specific anxiety and the stress of struggling with a handicapped child as shared by parents of retarded children.

Parents' Perception of Their Psychotic Child

A second line of formal investigation was carried out on another popular opinion. Clinicians have frequently expressed the belief that parents of psychotic children were perplexed in their communications (Meyers & Goldfarb, 1961) and emotionally handicapped in perceiving their child realistically. This position can be argued by pointing out that these parents cannot be too intellectually perplexed and emotionally cut off, since all their other children are usually normal. The psychodynamic clinician's response is to acknowledge these statistics, but then make the claim that a parent is probably different with each of his children. Nothing can therefore be inferred by the presence of normal children. We tried to evaluate this clinical argument by using more objective research methods (Schopler & Reichler, 1972).

Over 150 psychotic children had been seen over a seven-year period in our program, offering Developmental Therapy to psychotic children and their parents (Schopler & Reichler, 1971a). In this program parents worked as cotherapists on a reciprocal basis with the clinical staff. Over this period our staff had been impressed with the parents' intelligence and motivation to understand and to teach their own children. In this program structure, we simply did not encounter parental perplexity and emotional responses significantly different from staff perplexity and from staff responses. However, since this appraisal of parents was based on clinical impressions, we tested out formally at least one aspect of these impressions. That is, we tested the hypothesis that parents of psychotic children are able to estimate their child's level of functioning realistically and with reasonable accuracy. We asked parents to estimate their child's level of development in several areas. Their estimates were then compared with the results of standard psychological testing.

Parents were asked to make their estimates during the initial diagnostic interview, before any psychological testing was done. They were asked to estimate their psychotic child's level of functioning in years and months in the following six areas of development: (1) overall development, (2) language development, (3) motor development, (4) social age, (5) self-help sufficiency, and (6) mental development. Husbands made their estimates independently of their wives. Both of their estimates were compared with subsequent test results. These tests included the Vineland Social Maturity Scale, the Wechsler Intelligence Scale for Children, the Merrill-Palmer, the Bayley, and the Leiter International. No single intelligenence test could be used for all children, as some tests were limited by the age range covered and others by the child's limited understanding of the spoken word. Mental age was determined by the intelligence test most suitable for each child. This measure compared with parents' estimate of the child's general mental development. Although different tests were used, they were nevertheless rough indicators of general mental development and correlated significantly with social age from the Vineland Social Maturity Scale, $r = .83, p < .001$.

The correlational analysis between parent estimates and test results revealed significantly high correlations. These were subjected to further statistical analysis, involving control for the child's age and a comparison of differences in means of parent estimates. These analyses can be found in greater detail elsewhere (Schopler & Reichler, 1972) and are not elaborated here. However, in substance, we found that these parents were able to assess, quite accurately, their child's level of development in the six areas sampled by the study. This was consistent with the abilities of parents with retarded children to assess their children's current level of functioning (Wolfensberger & Kurtz, 1971). Although the entire parent group was good in assessing their children's developmental levels, there was a tendency for parents with mildly psychotic children to be relatively poorer estimators than were parents with severely psychotic children. A similar finding was reported for parents estimating the developmental levels of their retarded child (Heriot & Schmickel, 1967). In fact, the tendency for a mild handicap to produce greater mental stress than a severe handicap has been observed in other modalities. For example, the uncorrected inability to hear certain sound frequencies, which renders human conversation unintelligible for some partially deaf children, can produce more anxiety and tension than total deafness. Likewise, mild psychotic impairments involve functions which appear sufficiently close to normal, prompting a natural inclination by parents to push excessively both their perception of their child and his treatment, to try and get him into the normal range.

We found that the commonly held psychodynamic belief that parents of psychotic children have a uniquely distorted perception of their psychotic child, not necessarily bestowed on their other children, was not substantiated. On the contrary, as a group, these parents were able to assess their psychotic children's current developmental levels quite well.

However, we noted clinically that they have much greater difficulty knowing what to do and what to expect from this understanding. They appeared to be uncertain about its meaning for the child's future—what it means for his potential to achieve relative independence in his own life. Parental confusion about the child's future requires further research. We need to know what similar difficulties other people have in predicting a child's future development, including parents of normal children, and especially professionals charged with aiding parents in future planning. It is entirely possible that many professionals would not do better in trying to predict and plan for such a child's future. Those who base their predictions on unsubstantiated theories and beliefs would probably make misleading and incorrect recommendations in addition to the shared lack of certainty about optimum planning.

Future Trends Regarding Parents of Psychotic Children

There should be increased recognition that parents are more like the victims than the creators of their child's psychosis—that they are closer than anyone else to the child for helping with his survival rather than his destruction. With this understanding should also come some basic reorganization of approach. For the majority of psychotic or autistic children where neither specific causes nor specific treatment can be clearly established, the most important and primary question is, How are the most reasonable and rational decisions made for this child? Both diagnostic and treatment activities will be reorganized with this question in mind. Simultaneously, there may be a continued development of a variety of programs in recreation, special education, and vocational planning, so that future expectations will be easier to formulate and more reasonably humane living conditions will become available for every member of the family.

UNDERSTANDING AND TREATMENT OF PSYCHOTIC CHILDREN

A parent whose child shows psychotic or otherwise puzzling behavior has two major categories of special concern. The first has to do with trying to understand the child and his strange behavior. The second is the category of what to do about it, how to treat the child. These two areas of concern are intermingled with each other. Even when a parent is not inclined toward special attention and interest in human behavior, the psychotic child's lack or peculiarity of responsiveness fosters such interest. Likewise, the child's relatively limited response repertoire tends to produce many negative signals when the parent is acting on the basis of misunderstanding.

These children are more difficult to raise than normal children, even when there is no major misunderstanding about the child's development. However, when special child-rearing issues are compounded by major misapprehension and insecurity, the result is often psychotic and bizarre parent–child interactions. In the Developmental Therapy Program for psychotic children and their families, evolved by Robert J. Reichler and myself (Schopler & Reichler, 1971a), we have paid special attention to both categories of parental worry.

DIAGNOSTIC UNDERSTANDING

The next section covers a discussion of how parental misunderstanding of diagnosis and planning regarding their child is minimized in Developmental Therapy, followed by a discussion of how the treatment of the child is worked out.

What Is Wrong with the Child?

Although the children in our program come from the younger age range, most of our families have had several diagnostic evaluations for their child before they apply to our Center. If parents are well-off financially, their search for diagnostic clarity has often led them to centers all over the country. If their financial resources are in the average range, they have often been to various state and local agencies. Mental Health professionals have often referred to parents' effort to seek help in different agencies as "shopping," a kind of bargain hunting by self-centered and defensive people, unwilling to accept what they have been told. This attitude, as the reader may now anticipate, derives from certain absolute and ill-fitting myth-belief systems of the past. It is true that a parent's repeated trips to different diagnostic centers—seeking answers to issues involving their psychotic child's survival—bears some resemblance to a woman's unending search for the right party dress. However, a closer look can reveal the other side to this simile.

Often the parents' confusion has increased with each evaluation. A far too common source of the confusion has been that the findings and opinions of the results have been withheld. Records and charts are stamped "Confidential." This usually means confidential from parents. Reasons for such secrecy are variable. However, they usually include some of the following aspects: The entire evaluation was written up as a psychodynamic account of family personalities and how their interaction produced an autistic child. Had these findings been shared with the parents, the information would not have answered the questions they were faced with and often the findings contained major errors. Sometimes there is ambiguous neurological evidence for brain damage, and unclear psychological testing for evidence of mental retardation. The confidentiality of the records then becomes an effort to shield parents from uncertainties and the shock of unpleasant possibilities. For the diagnostic evaluation in our Program, we take the position that the daily life and uncertainties of knowledge about autistic children are both sufficiently and realistically great, that they should not be confounded with self-protecting professionalism.

Records and charts are not kept secret from parents. IQ scores are not kept as classified information. How they are derived and their limitations and use are briefly explained. In a similar fashion the limitations of neurological tests, still largely based on the neurological assessment of adults, are reviewed. The existing absence of diagnostic precision is acknowledged, including the fact that because a child may be considered autistic or psychotic, does not mean that he may not also be brain damaged and retarded. We do not withhold from parents our clinical impressions regarding a child with the kind of language impairment characterizing most autistic children. That is, we have not yet been able to uncover clinical evidence that the effect of child-rearing practices could have been the source of this kind of language impairment. In short, our experience has been that parents' shock at unpleasant information or lack of clear knowledge was never as great as the confusion resulting from professional attempts to protect them from both.

How to Plan for the Child

For parents, specific test results and diagnostic formulations are often less important than what these tests and conclusions mean for both their long- and short-range planning. Many diagnostic centers, on the other hand, see their main function as doing extensive evaluations, leaving the planning to some other agency. If, in addition to not offering specific practical advice, the diagnostic results are interpreted with a term such as emotionally disturbed, the implied recommendations are usually vague and distressing. Many people construe emotionally disturbed to mean that the child is reacting to some sort of traumatic family interaction. The trauma is generally not well-defined nor is the resolution to its effects. Parents usually leave this sort of evaluation more incapacitated in their abilities to plan rationally than before the study was undertaken.

In the Developmental Therapy program, parents' long-range plans for their child are discussed by sharing frankly with them prognostic probabilities based on research findings. The best indicators for long-range expectations for the young psychotic child at this time appears still to be his IQ score (Gittelman & Birch, 1967). The child with an IQ of under 50 tends to remain quite stable over time. Those with higher IQs tend to be more variable depending on education and experience. Parents often need to know these kinds of probabilities in order to arrange their limited resources for the needs of all the family members.

If a child's psychosis also includes severe retardation, the degree of independence he can be expected to reach is severely limited. Parents of such a child may have to struggle less with whether to place the child in an institution, as with the issue of when to place him. Regardless of these long-range concerns, parents usually have pressing questions on how to manage the child's difficult behavior now and what the best methods for teaching him might be.

Immediate Problems of Adjustment and Learning

For a psychotic child, a significant number of his behavior problems is usually closely related to the peculiarities of his learning channels, and his inabilities to comprehend his environment. For example, some psychotic children perceive and learn more through their visual modalities than through their hearing. Such a child often experiences displeasure or punishment from adults who find him unresponsive to their verbal directions. The child's peculiarities of learning are sometimes subtle and difficult to detect. However, the resulting autistic symptom, such as "avoiding eye contact" is recognized more easily.

The diagnostic evaluation in our Program is designed to clarify both the child's developmental levels, peculiarities of learning, and signs of psychosis. A psychoeducational profile was developed through which various learning functions could be sampled in the younger child. The purpose of this test was not to obtain an IQ score, but instead to see how a child responded to tasks, sampling several areas of learning. The system of scoring the child's responses was designed to outline an educational profile to be used for initial identification of the child's individual special education needs.

The child's response to each task is scored according to one of three ratings. It is scored 0 if he shows no understanding of the task or makes no response. The response is scored 2 if it is correct. It is scored 1 if partially correct or showing some emerging understanding of the task requirements. A score of 0 usually indicates that the task is too far beyond the child's comprehension to make a current target for special educational effort. The correct response shows already established skills, but they may need exercise in variations of similar problems. However, it is this emerging comprehension of the task which forms the main direction for the child's educational program.

The individual items on this Profile were based on experience with tasks and learning difficulties characteristic of autistic or psychotic children. They include the areas of imitation both vocally and motorically; perceptual discriminations in the visual and auditory modalities; gross and fine motor skills and the ability to integrate visual information with motoric behavior; language; and cognitive functions. The items in these areas are arrayed according to developmental complexity based on normal children's responses. There are also pathology ratings which simply indicate the presence and absence of abnormal behavior. These are used for assessing the degree of psychosis and programming for reduction of psychosis.

Parents' observation and firsthand knowledge of these assessment procedures form a substantial basis for managing and interacting more successfully with their psychotic child. Paradoxical to the aims of some other psychotherapies, parents become more, rather than less, self-conscious of their responses to their child as they understand him more objectively. This is necessary because spontaneous responses to normal child-rearing issues are not adequate for many problems of psychotic children. As parents become more conscious of these needs they can often interact with more pleasure and spontaneity toward their autistic child.

So far, the discussion of treatment has focused on helping parents observe and attend to their child, to become aware of his special education needs. The next section is concerned with how that understanding is converted into management and teaching in Developmental Therapy.

THERAPEUTIC TREATMENT

Autistic or psychotic children have been exposed to a remarkable array of therapies during the past three decades. The list includes nonexclusively electroconvulsive shock, residential treatment or custodial isolation, psychoanalytic play therapy and group therapy, electronic typewriters, operant conditioning, drug and megavitamin therapy. Proponents of each new therapy have enthusiastically reported success, limited in degree to only some of the children in each program. However, we are not able to answer such basic questions as, Is the child who responds best to one treatment also most likely to do well in some of the others? Conversely, will the child with the worst progress in one treatment be likely to have the worst in others? The criteria and duration of success have been sufficiently variable that there has scarcely been any consensus on what constituted the treatment of choice.

Because of these conditions, in our Developmental Therapy Program, the current state of the art is frankly acknowledged with the parents. Working collaboratively with the staff, parents are taught to function as cotherapists with their own psychotic child. To this collaboration parents contribute their unique expertise on their own child, an expertise consisting of their long-term observations, their unique motivation for raising their own child, and their interest in living with less rather than more stress at home. The staff's main contribution to the collaboration derives from experience with many such children, motivation to work with this group of youngsters, and familiarity with current research and knowledge.

Developmental Concept

Although individualization of educational program for each child and family is basic to effective help, the structure of developmental therapy also offers explicit direction for the process. The concept of development is emphasized as a reminder that children, normal or otherwise, change with age, more than adults. Furthermore, various functions within the same child can be understood operating on different developmental levels. Appropriate adult responses can often be best approximated from the normal response to a particular developmental level. For example, a five-year-old autistic child may have the motor coordination of a normal five-year-old, but a language level of a two-year-old. While he could be taught to use a tricycle, this might best be done using simple speech appropriate to the two-year level. This is not to say that autistic children or their behaviors are just like normal behaviors of younger children. It is, however, to say that one of the soundest bridges to the special understanding of autistic children is across their similarities and common needs with younger children.

Treatment Structure

In addition to learning a developmental perspective, many parents must unlearn some of the child-rearing myths that they have been taught. Some of these came directly from mental health professionals. Having been told that their child was emotionally disturbed, parents were often led to believe that the child would be helped by expressing himself freely and with a minimum of restraints. Parents' fear of harming their child by expecting him to act within the confines of family life often paralyzed any effective disciplinary efforts. Our clinical work with autistic children, on the contrary, had indicated that these children responded more constructively to a structured learning situation.

We conducted a controlled study on the question of structure to test these child-rearing beliefs against experimental data. The children included in the study were exposed to a relatively unstructured program for two weeks, and then the cycle was repeated for another two weeks each of the structured and unstructured sessions. A structured session was defined as one in which the adult determined what material was to be worked with, for how long the child was to work with it, and the manner in which he was to work. The unstructured session, on the other hand, was defined as one in which the child selected the material, decided how long to work with it, and the manner in which he would use it. The same materials were used for each child over the period of study, but materials differed among children according to what was most appropriate for each one.

The therapy sessions were observed through a one-way mirror and rated by three observers. A time sampling procedure was used in which the following five variables were rated: (1) attending versus not attending, (2) affect— appropriate versus inappropriate, (3) relatedness versus not relating, (4) meaningful versus nonmeaningful vocalization, and (5) psychotic versus nonpsychotic behavior. Reliability studies between raters showed satisfactory levels of agreement. The ratings of the children on these five variables were repeated under each structured and unstructured condition. The analyses of these data were reported in detail elsewhere (Schopler et al., 1971). However, the results showed clear trends that these psychotic children learned more adaptive behavior and related more appropriately to adults during the structured than the unstructured situations. They also showed less psychotic behavior during the structured sessions than the unstructured ones.

Although the children as a group tended to respond more appropriately under the structured conditions, there were significant differences among the individual children's responses to the change in condition. Further analysis of individual variations showed that the key factor in the child's response to the changes in structure related to differences in the child's response to the changes in structure related to differences in the children's developmental levels. That is, the children who were ranked higher developmentally according to their social age on the Vineland Social Maturity Scale and according to staff ratings were better able to handle the unstructured condition, while children who ranked lower developmentally were less able to handle the unstructured situations and responded more favorably to the structured.

The implications of this study for therapy and education were consistent with our clinical impressions. That is, psychotic or autistic children's favorable response to structure suggested that the relatively unstructured psychoanalytic play therapy was not an appropriate treatment for them. Moreover, the type and degree of structure should be regulated according to the individual child and his various levels of function, as might be determined by the Psychoeducational Profile discussed above. A highly structured treatment technique, such as operant conditioning, especially when applied rigidly from a laboratory model of learning, will not offer maximum help for an autistic child, especially when the rates and levels of development in more than one behavior unit are disregarded (Lovaas, 1973).

Both the data from this study and clinical experience contributed to our belief that the optimum learning situation for autistic children, as for others, was one which has more external structure for acquiring new learning patterns or those involving the child's more specific handicap. On the other hand, while practicing those patterns which have already been mastered and internalized, the child may make better use of freedom from external structure.

Cotherapy Treatment Procedure

Parents are usually able to understand the developmental structure quite readily. Within this framework therapy objectives may be considered in two interdependent categories. These include behavior management and special education procedures. Behavior problems may involve temper tantrums or toilet training difficulties and others which mainly appear in the home rather than during visits to the Center. In collaboration with the parents, the problem is broken down into the most manageable units. Whenever possible, coping techniques are demonstrated by the staff before parents are requested to carry them out at home. Depending on the child, developmental readiness, and degree of handicap, some aspects of the behavior problem may be handled with intensive persistence while others involve acceptance of handicap and slow learning.

The special education procedures are centered around preschool skills and worked out directly with the child during his weekly visits. Parents observe therapist's demonstrations, participate in working out a home program for their child, and work with him in daily sessions. The specific approaches developed in these home programs determine the child's success during the sessions and also the parents' satisfaction with their interaction at home. A more detailed description of the program structure for working collaboratively with parents has been described elsewhere (Schopler & Reichler, 1971b). However, we have found that the best behavior management techniques and special education methods can prove ineffective or fail if certain conditions of trust and care do not exist between parents and staff members. Those conditions are difficult to specify. However, four components of this relationship can be identified and expressed in administrative policy and structure.

Frank Sharing of Information

We have already discussed the parental confusion and demoralization that can result from keeping diagnostic information or ignorance confidential and secret from them. Regardless of the professional's motive, whether to protect the child, the parent, or the staff, the outcome tends to be counterproductive. In a similar vein, admonitions and efforts to prevent parents from reading the professional literature is equally undesirable. There is not enough known about the causes, the diagnosis, and the treatment of severely disturbed children to justify such paternalistically protective efforts. There is still too little agreement among clinicians and researchers, and there are still too many experimental efforts mistaken as panaceas to justify any meaningful censorship of reading. If, on the other hand, both the existence and the absence of available information and research is jointly explored and evaluated by staff and parents, the probability of increased emotional disturbance for both parents and children can usually be avoided or diminished.

Definition of Therapist Role

Our therapists' role is defined by the dual functions of child therapist and parent consultant. As a child therapist the work is confined to evaluating and working with the child directly, demonstrating and modeling useful approaches to the participating parent. As a parent consultant, the working space is on the observation side of the one-way mirror. The consultant helps to direct the parents' attention to the relevant part of the demonstration and discusses all other questions and problems parents may raise in connection with their handicapped child. All staff members are required to work in both of these roles. This helps them to become familiar with both child and parent side of the interaction and avoids overidentification with either side. In the traditional mental health team usually the psychiatrist saw the child, the psychologist made assessments, and the social worker saw the parents. This arrangement made for status priorities unwarranted by the problems and reduced clarity and directness of communication.

We have also found distinct advantages to both children and their parents when the therapists who work with them were "paraprofessionals" or intelligent and experienced laymen rather than highly trained and specialized professionals. Often the specialized professional, whether psychiatrist, psychologist, teacher, or speech therapist, has certain skills and professional sets which make him respond more in terms of his specialized knowledge than to the needs of the individual child. Some of our most effective therapists have come from various educational backgrounds including Chinese history, linguistics, education, and art. The diffusion of professional lines promotes the climate for an effective working relationship because: (1) it structures concern with the needs of the individual child and the particular family rather than with a special professional point of view; (2) the therapists share the responsibility with the parents for selecting the most useful special technique to fit their individual situation; and (3) since the children are a heterogeneous group and no single treatment has yet been established for the entire group, the nonspecialized therapist best fits the current state of knowledge about childhood psychosis.

Relativity of Behavior Modification Techniques

We have operated on the assumption that the most effective behavior management techniques are not established as "scientifically true," but vary significantly from family to family. Many psychologists have reported dramatic success in shaping the behaviors of autistic or psychotic children. These reports often originate from the controlled environment of an institution or a psychology laboratory. It is tempting to consider these techniques as scientifically established and to pass them on as such to parents. If the technique does not then work in the home, the fault can be blamed on the parental environment. We have found that parent–child–staff relations are maintained at the most productive level when behavioral management techniques are selected relative to their suitability in the individual situation. A technique may be correct and effective in an artifically controlled environment and ineffective or incorrect in a free home environment.

Parental Authority and Responsibility

Perhaps the most important of these four aspects of a good working relationship is the recognition that parents are responsible for their children and are the most likely people to have their children's well-being at heart. Especially with young and unusual children like the psychotic, parents are the most likely people to become experts on the peculiar learning patterns of their own child. They are the most likely people to have the investment and commitment to help the child maximize his potential, however limited. This recognition is sometimes difficult to maintain when parents are confused and distraught by their child to the point of considering institutional placement. At those times it is easy to see parents as rejecting and incompetent. However, in most cases, parents are reacting to the stress produced by the difficulties of the psychotic child on all the family members, rather than abdicating their parental responsibility. There are no clear criteria for when a child needs to be institutionalized. Sometimes, especially when there is also severe retardation, the child will need institutional care, and it is mainly a question of timing. The answer to this question depends on the resources of both the family and the community. When parents' authority is maintained and they are helped with their difficulties, we have found that they usually evaluate their child realistically, making substantial efforts in his behalf, institutionalizing when necessary, and electing to keep their child at home in the vast majority of cases.

Summary and Projection of Treatment Trends

In the past, some key theories about autism were locked to the prescribed therapy for their verification. For example, some residential treatment (Bettelheim, 1967) involved separating the child indefinitely from his parents and replacing them with professional parent surrogates. This parentectomy therapy and the psychogenic theories were often presented as evidence of one for the other. A similar relationship was argued between learning theory and operant conditioning. Many therapists assumed that any desirable behavior could be shaped if the right reinforcement contingencies were found. Ferster (1961) confirmed this view by proposing that autistic behavior was caused by parental inability to provide a proper reinforcement history for the child. Such circular reasoning is not the link between the theoretical assumptions or research and Developmental Therapy. Although the effectiveness of this treatment approach may lend support to the related theoretical positions, we expect future research to supply the sound basis for revision and change in optimum therapy.

Future improvement in the treatment of autistic or psychotic children will also depend on research. Research into underlying causes can be expected to provide some answers. In the past, the aims and methods of research have often run against the aims and methods of treatment. This resulted in lack of relevance in research and lack of necessary research cooperation from treatment programs. This conflict may be accepted and understood better as the collaboration becomes more successful. With better understanding of the biological bases of the handicapping conditions, better recognition of subgroups within the broad category of childhood psychosis should develop. Some of these may have their handicap neutralized through biochemical and dietary interventions. Other subgroups involving accidents of prenatal care and genetic aberrations may be prevented. However, many of these children, regardless of the origins of their handicap, need better special education and social support expressed through special environmental considerations. This latter need may turn out to be the more important in the long run. It may also be the most difficult since man's humanity towards his fellow has not always improved with scientific progress.

RESEARCH AND SOCIAL ACTION

Often research in social science runs against powerful political forces. The successful overcoming of this conflict characterizes the current trends with autistic children. Historically, myths of psychoanalytic theory and extremes of environmentalism identified parents as the primary causal agents in their child's psychotic development. At the same time parents were unable to organize the kind of social support for their children as had parents of retarded children. Not until the publication of Rimland's (1964) scholarly review of the literature on autism was a widely circulated refutation of the psychogenic position available. It was no accident that Rimland was instrumental in organizing the National Society for Autistic Children. This Society, composed mainly of parents with autistic children, has recognized that one of the most unnecessary sources of suffering for families with autistic children was both the misinformation about the disorder and unavailability of community resources. Accordingly, the organization has dedicated itself to supporting both educational services and research on autism and related childhood disorders. It has made some major strides toward the attainment of these goals on both federal and state levels.

One of the noteworthy examples of what local efforts can accomplish can be illustrated by the activities of the North Carolina Chapter of the National Society for Austic Children. Using the Development Therapy approach of collaboration with professionals, they promoted legislative support for a statewide extension of the Developmental Therapy Program described above. Under the title of Division for the Treatment and Education of Autistic and Related Communications Handicapped Children (TEACCH), a state program was mandated in the Department of Psychiatry of the University of North Carolina School of Medicine. The legislation called for three Developmental Therapy Centers in the eastern, western, and central areas of the State, with special education classes in the Program, but located in the public schools.

Both parents and program staff participated in working toward integrating the child's learning experiences at home, via the Centers, with those of the school. Specialized help in speech pathology and medical services was made available to the families. Not only did parents function as cotherapists for their children but also the legislation allowed for their participation in the classroom, when feasible. The special education needs for these children are as variable as their handicaps and developmental levels. Likewise, there are differences between the eastern coastal area, the central piedmont, and the western mountain country. Variations in special education experiments in different classrooms reflected these regional differences. For example, some schools helped with the special transportation problems of these youngsters when the state had not done so; some were flexible in moving a child from special education to the normal classes as needed; others have developed a program of social interaction between normal and handicapped children. No claims for the one best special education technique has yet been published. However, the humanizing effects of the interaction between the psychotic children, their peers, and parents have become evident.

Summer Camp

Parents have cooperatively established a free summer camp program for their autistic children. The pleasurable and constructive response to the camp experience by the children is reflected in staff enthusiasm and growth of the camp program. The parents' group is currently planning to stimulate other camp programs throughout the state to enable children to remain within reasonable proximity of their homes.

The absence of camp fees did not mean absence of cost. It was interesting to see how parents have been meeting camp expenses. Depending on the skills and interests of individual parents, funds were raised by organizing art auctions, special theatre and film events, cooky sales, turkey shoots, and other fund raising efforts. For their camp counselors and aides, they have recruited enthusiastic young graduate students in education, medicine, psychology, and other behavioral sciences.

CONCLUSION

This chapter attempted to trace out some misconceptions, blind beliefs, and biases from the past about autism or psychotic children. Changes in these past attitudes were suggested in the light of current clinical experience and research. These changes have affected the diagnostic grouping of children, the study of causative factors, and the treatment of psychotic children and their parents.

It is worthwhile to note that both errors of generalizing beyond data and excessive pride in one's own observations and conclusions are more easily repeated than avoided. Openness to new clinical data and research findings offer a fragile safeguard against using social science concepts beyond their social relevancies. This openness is also the basis for keeping in meaningful interdependence what can be known about these children, scientifically and objectively, and what the social resources, values, and desires for them may be.

Future research will probably reveal new subgroups of children within the category of childhood psychosis. These new groupings may be defined by specific metabolic, biochemical, and brain abnormalities. This may mean greater improvement in adaptation for some children than we are now able to achieve. And perhaps even more important, there will be greater acceptance of aberration and handicap in a small percentage of children.

A society worthy of its name mobilizes the desire to enable these children and their families to live a reasonably dignified life. It also finds the capacity to provide the special education, services and environmental support to approximate the realization of this intent.

REFERENCES

Alpern, G. Measurement of "untestable" autistic children. *Journal of Abnormal Psychology*, 1967, **12**, 16–25.

Allport, G. W. *ABC's of scapegoating*. Anti-Defamation League, 1966.

Bender, L. Childhood schizophrenia. *Psychiatric Quarterly*, 1953, **27**, 663–81.

Bettelheim, B. Feral children and autistic children. *American Journal of Sociology*, 1959, **64**, 455–67.

Bettelheim, B. *The empty fortress*. New York: Macmillan, 1967.

Creak, M. Schizophrenic syndrome in childhood: Further progress report of a working party. *Developmental Medicine and Child Neurology*, 1964, **6**, 530–535

Eberhardy, F. The view from the couch. *Journal of Child Psychology and Psychiatry*, 1967, **8**, 257–63.

Ekstein, R., & Wallerstein, J. Observations on the psychology of borderline and psychotic children. *Psychoanalytic study of the child*. Vol. 9. New York: International Universities Press, 1954.

Ferster, C. B. Positive reinforcement and behavioral deficits of autistic children. *Child Development*, 1961, **32**, 437.

Gesell, A. *Wolf child and human child*. New York: Harper, 1941.

Gittelman, M., & Birch, H. G. Childhood schizophrenia: Intellect, neurologic status, perinatal risk, prognosis, and family pathology. *Archives of General Psychiatry*, 1967, **17**, 16.

Goldfarb, W. Receptor preferences in schizophrenic children. *Archives of Neurology and Psychiatry*, 1956, **76**, 643–652.

Heriot, J. T., & Schmickel, C. A. Maternal estimate of I.Q. in children evaluated for learning potential. *American Journal of Mental Deficiency*, 1967, **71**, 920–924.

Kanner, L. Autistic disturbances of affective contact. *Nervous Child*, 1943, **2**, 217.

Kanner, L. Problems of nosology and psychodynamics in early infantile autism. *American Journal of Orthopsychiatry*, 1949, **19**, 416–426.

Kysar, J. The two camps in child psychiatry: A report from a psychiatrist-father of an autistic and retarded child. *American Journal of Psychiatry*, 1968, **125**, 103.

Lidz, T. Intrafamilial environment of the schizophrenic patient: VI The transmission of irrationality. *Archives of General Psychiatry*, 1958, **79**, 305–316.

Lovaas, O. I., Koegel, R., Simmons, J. Q., & Stevens, J. Some generalization and follow-up measures on autistic children in behavior therapy. *Journal of Applied Behavior Analysis*, 1973, **6**, 131–166.

Lovibond, S. H. The object sorting test and conceptual thinking in schizophrenia. *Austalian Journal of Psychiatry*, 1954, **6**, 52.

Mahler, M. On child psychosis and schizophrenia. Autistic and symbotic infantile psychoses. *Psychoanalytic study of the child*. Vol. 7. New York: International Universities Press, 1952.

Meyers, D. I., & Goldfarb, W. Studies of perplexity in mothers of schizophrenic children. *American Journal of Orthopsychiatry*, 1961, **31**, 551.

Ornitz, E. M. Childhood autism: A review of the clinical and experimental literature. *California Medicine*, 1973, **118**, 29–47.

Ornitz, E. M., & Ritvo, E. R. Perceptual inconstancy in early infantile autism. *Archives of General Psychiatry*, 1968, **18**, 79.

Park, C. *The siege*. New York: Harcourt, Brace & World, 1967.

Pitfield, M., & Oppenheim, A. Child rearing attitudes of mothers of psychotic children. *Journal of Child Psychology and Psychiatry*, 1964, **1**, 51–57.

Rank, B. Adaptation of the psychoanalytic technique for the treatment of young children with atypical development. *American Journal of Orthopsychiatry*, 1949, **19**, 130.

Reichler, R. J., & Schopler, E. Observations on the nature of human relatedness. *Journal of Autism and Childhood Schizophrenia*, 1971, **1**, 283–296.

Rimland, B. *Infantile autism*. New York: Appleton-Century-Crofts, 1964.

Rutter, M. Concepts of autism: A review of research. *Journal of Child Psychology and Psychiatry*, 1968, **9**, 1.

Rutter, M. Childhood schizophrenia reconsidered. *Journal of Autism and Childhood Schizophrenia*, 1972, **2**, (4), 315.

Schopler, E. Early infantile autism and sensory processes. *Archives of General Psychiatry*, 1965, **13**, 327–335.

Schopler, E. Visual versus tactual receptor preferences in normal and schizophrenic children. *Journal of Abnormal Psychology*, 1966, **71**, 108.

Schopler, E. Parents of psychotic children as scapegoats. *Journal of Contemporary Psychotherapy*, 1971, **4**, 17–22.

Schopler, E., Brehm, S., Kinsbourne, M., & Reichler, R. J. Effect of treatment structure on development in autistic children. *Archives of General Psychiatry,* 1971, **24,** 415–421.

Schopler, E., & Loftin, J. Thought disorders in parents of psychotic children: A function of test anxiety. *Archives General Psychiatry,* 1969, **20,** 174.

Schopler, E., & Reichler, R. J. Developmental progress of a psychotic child over a three-year period. Film produced by Child Research Project, University of North Carolina, Chapel Hill, North Carolina, 1969.

Schopler, E., & Reichler, R. J. Developmental therapy by parents with their own psychotic child. In M. Rutter (Ed.), *Infantile autism: Concepts, characteristics and treatment.* London: Churchill Livingston, 1971. Pp. 206–227. (a)

Schopler, E., & Reichler, R. J. Parents as cotherapists in the treatment of psychotic children. *Journal of Autism and Childhood Schizophrenia,* 1971, **1,** 87–102. (b)

Schopler, E., & Reichler, R. J. How well do parents understand their own psychotic child? *Journal of Autism and Childhood Schizophrenia,* 1972, **2,** 387–400.

Singer, M., & Wynne, L. Thought disorder and family relations of schizophrenics. *Archives of General Psychiatry,* 1965, **12,** 201–212.

Wild, C. Disturbed styles of thinking: Implications of disturbed styles of thinking manifested on the object sorting test by the parents of schizophrenic patients. *Archives of General Psychiatry,* 1965, **13,** 464–470.

Wing, L. *Autistic children.* New York: Drummer, Magel, 1972.

Wolfensberger, W., & Kurtz, R. A. Measurement of parents' perception of their children's development. *Genetic Psychology Monographs,* 1971, **83,** 3–92.

Index